Violence and Health Care Profession

Edited by

Til Wykes

Department of Psychology
Institute of Psychiatry
Maudsley Hospital
London, UK

CHAPMAN & HALL

London · Glasgow · Weinheim · New York · Tokyo · Melbourne · Madras

Published by Chapman & Hall, 2–6 Boundary Row, London SE1 8HN, UK

Chapman & Hall, 2–6 Boundary Row, London SE1 8HN, UK

Blackie Academic & Professional, Wester Cleddens Road, Bishopbriggs, Glasgow G64 2NZ, UK

Chapman & Hall GmbH, Pappelallee 3, 69469 Weinheim, Germany

Chapman & Hall Inc., One Penn Plaza, 41st Floor, New York NY 10119, USA

Chapman & Hall Japan, Thomson Publishing Japan, Hirakawacho Nemoto Building, 6F, 1-7-11 Hirakawa-cho, Chiyoda-ku, Tokyo 102, Japan

Chapman & Hall Australia, Thomas Nelson Australia, 102 Dodds Street, South Melbourne, Victoria 3205, Australia

Chapman & Hall India, R. Seshadri, 32 Second Main Road, CIT East, Madras 600 035, India

Distributed in the USA and Canada by Singular Publishing Group Inc., 4284 41st Street, San Diego, California 92105

First edition 1994

© 1994 Chapman & Hall

Typeset in 10/12 Palatino by Mews Photosetting, Beckenham, Kent
Printed in Great Britain by
St Edmundsbury Press Ltd, Bury St Edmunds, Suffolk

ISBN 0 412 46170 6   1 56593 132 7 (USA)

A catalogue record for this book is available from the British Library

Library of Congress Catalog Card Number: 93-74877

Contents

Contributors

Stanley Bute
Formerly Social Work Manager, Hampshire Social Services, Julian House, Roman Drive, Chilworth, Southampton, SO1 7HS.

R.L. Dearden
Department of Nursing Studies, University of Birmingham, Birmingham, B15 2TT.

Anne Greaves
Health and Safety Officer, NALGO (now UNISON), 1 Mabledon Place, London, WC1H 9AJ.

F.D. Richard Hobbs
Professor, Department of General Practice, University of Birmingham, Birmingham, B15 2TT.

Andrew McDonnell
School of Psychology, University of Birmingham, Birmingham, B15 2TT.

John McEvoy
Solihull Healthcare, Berwicks Lane, Marston Green, Birmingham, B37 7XR.

Colin MacKay
Health and Safety Executive, Human Factors Division, Room 251, Magdalen House, Stanley Precinct, Bootle, Merseyside, L20 1QZ.

Gillian Mezey
Consultant Psychiatrist and Honorary Senior Lecturer, Forensic Psychiatry Department, St Georges Hospital Medical School, London, SW17 0RE.

David Miers
Professor and Director, Centre for Professional Legal Studies, Cardiff Law School, University of Wales, PO Box 427, Cardiff, CF1 1XD.

Lyn Pilowsky
Wellcome Research Fellow and Honorary Lecturer, Department of Psychology, Institute of Psychiatry, De Crespigny Park, London, SE5 8AF.

Dr J. Shapland
Faculty of Law, University of Sheffield, Crookes Moore Building, Sheffield, S10 1FL.

Richard Whittington
Lecturer, Department of Health and Community Studies, Chester College, Cheyney Road, Chester, CH1 4BJ.

Til Wykes
Consultant Clinical Psychologist and Senior Lecturer, Department of Psychology, Institute of Psychiatry, De Crespigny Park, London, SE5 8AF.

Introduction

Til Wykes

BACKGROUND

The recent publication of several surveys on violence was the impetus
for this book. The first was carried out in 1986 by the Health and Safety
Commission Health Services Advisory Committee (1987). They
conducted a comprehensive survey of the incidence of violence to 5000
workers in five separate health districts. The results from the 3000
people who eventually replied made many in the caring professions
worried. One in 200 workers had suffered a major injury following
a violent attack during the previous year and a further one in ten
needed first aid following an assault. Other surveys also showed high
risks: of social service staff, 6% had suffered an attack in the past 5
years (Saunders, 1987), and social workers were at even higher risk.
29% had been assaulted in the last 3 years (Rowett, 1986). In addition,
4% of general practitioners had experienced an attack resulting in injury
in the past year (D'Urso and Hobbs, 1989). Clinical psychologists were
also at risk – 53% had been assaulted at least once during their
professional career and 18% in the past year (Perkins, 1991).

Media reports of extreme violence seem to be the tip of the iceberg.
Many staff are attacked and some of these attacks have serious physical
or psychological consequences that interfere with the victim's ability
to return to their full working capacity. This loss of highly trained
staff should be recognized by employers and the community. Not
only are they a scarce resource but the cost of training is extremely
high.

Is the violence increasing?

It is not clear whether the problem of violence has increased or whether
there is now more concern and less tolerance of its effects. Longitudinal
data are scarce but information from health authorities suggests
that the number of incidents has increased and data from a violence

register at a psychiatric hospital in London has shown a three-fold increase in violence over ten years (Noble and Rodger, 1989).

Why should the violence increase?

Apart from the increase in violence in the community there are also changes in the way services are provided that may also increase both the likelihood and the severity of the effects of assaults. More people work in the community, visiting people in their own homes or working in geographically isolated sites or after hours so there is less chance that they can call on assistance when difficult situations have arisen.

Some professions involved with health care have also gained more legal powers over their clients' affairs. Some have control over parts of their income (e.g. the social fund, signing sick notes, etc.). Others have powers to take children into care and to commit people to a mental hospital. These social controls will obviously, on occasion, bring them into conflict.

Also, members of the caring professions have many stresses to face during the course of their work. They care for people in distress, and work unsociable and long hours, often receiving poor pay and working conditions. This background level of stress affects the worker's ability to perceive and to communicate effectively when threats arise, hence there is an escalation of an incident.

What are the effects on staff?

Apart from the risk of violence that health care professionals are under by the nature of their work, there are particular difficulties specific to their roles as carers – the people who assault them are often the very people who they are caring for. Few other professions apart from prison officers, police officers and teachers are in this position. Health professionals are often expected to face their assailants and even to continue to provide a service to them following an attack. These factors are likely to affect the victim's ability to cope with the psychological consequences of threats and assaults.

THE SCOPE OF THIS BOOK

Violence in the course of a health professional's work has been highlighted by the media reports of the killings of social workers, doctors and nurses over the last 10 years. However, these gruesome reports do not address important issues about violence and have left health care professionals uncertain about how to weigh the risks.

This book aims to fill this gap by providing information that, where possible, is backed up by sound empirical data. Research relevant to this area is relatively unsystematized, so findings from other areas are borrowed where relevant. Despite the disorganization of the research effort there are examples of good practice in health and social services. These will be highlighted where appropriate even though their efficacy may not yet have been evaluated.

No two groups of workers are under similar risks so as many kinds of occupation and work patterns are covered as possible given the space restrictions.

The information will include:

- the risks that different groups of workers are under so that they can make informed decisions about their work patterns;
- how to assess the risks for particular individuals and situations;
- what sort of physical and psychological consequences to expect after being involved in an incident as well as how to claim compensation;
- some guidelines for the prevention and management of violence; and
- how to implement changes in an organization that will improve safety.

DEFINING VIOLENCE

The major barrier to further scientific and practical progress on violence at work is the lack of accepted definitions. Serious violence noted on violent incidence forms or in research papers may not represent the same physical severity. Some studies include threatened violence whose severity is assessed by putative victims whereas others only investigate actual physical harm. What is needed is a definition that is easy to understand and has little ambiguity. It also needs to cover the wide range of violent situations faced by health service staff, the majority of which are not life-threatening. The definition given below tries to achieve these goals. It is similar to the ones used in the major research studies and if it were to be adopted by violence researchers and health service bodies to collect future data this would be a significant success.

Violence may be defined as follows:

- **Physical assault**: an assault with or without a weapon which results in actual physical harm, for instance bruising or lacerations. This includes sexual assaults.
- **Physical abuse**: attempted assault that did not result in actual harm.

- **Threats**: verbal or written threats that suggest harm to a person or property. This category includes sexual harassment or other forms of inappropriate sexual behaviour.
- **Damage to property** belonging to a person or organization.

Sexual assaults and harassment are included with other forms of violence in the above definitions. However, in recognition of some of the specific issues that should be addressed in this area there is a separate chapter devoted to this topic in this book.

As well as a definition to describe incidents there also needs to be an agreed framework to describe assailants. One possibility is to describe them in the following way:

- **Direct user of service**: where the assailant is in current receipt of a service provided by the health care professional at the time of the incident, i.e. the assailant could be described as a patient, client or user;
- **Indirect user of service**: where the assailant is closely associated with a current user (relative, friend, etc.) of the service;
- **No current user of service**: where the assailant does not receive the health care service and is not closely associated with a user of the service.

This sort of definition would allow the monitoring of the increase of incidents for health care professionals. For instance, if there were an increasing number of violent incidents for social workers it would be possible to attribute this either to structural changes in their jobs, for example, their increasing role as gatekeepers of services and resources, or to increases in violent crime generally. When mental health care workers are moving their work base into the community it will be important to identify whether any increases in incidents might be attributed to the increasing severity of disability in their clients as access to hospital services declines or whether it is the result of changes in job location so that staff are working in more dangerous areas.

Terminology

Throughout this book the term 'victim' has been used to refer to the person who is assaulted or threatened with violence. Although there are some drawbacks, the author has found it difficult to find a replacement since it provides a factual description of the position of health care practitioners who are faced with violence in the course of their work. The author also considers it to be helpful for staff to realize that they have much in common with people who are the victims of threats or assaults in the community and who would normally be sanctioned by society as having a legitimate claim to compensation, social support and counselling.

Victims are normal people who are thrown off balance by abnormal events. They are at risk of physical and emotional illness. They respond well to support and eventually may be able to consider themselves as survivors.

A caution It is important that professionals should know the actual risk and be aware of how sensitization to violence may occur through the sensationalizing of particular incidents. Not all health care professionals will be involved in a violent incident. However, knowing the actual risks and the factors leading up to incidents will not prevent them all and practitioners need to be aware that the responsibility for violence lies clearly with the perpetrator.

The chapters in this book were designed to cover all aspects of the problem of violence for health care workers; nevertheless, each chapter may be read in isolation as a reference text. It is in order to make each one comprehensive that some overlap may exist and apologies are made to those who wish to read the book from cover to cover.

WHO SHOULD READ THIS BOOK?

Any health care professional who wishes to know the risks and effects of violent incidents in the course of their work should read this book. In addition, anyone who is at risk of violence during the course of their work might also be interested in the chapters on how to assess risks and what sort of effects to expect as a victim. Workers who are acknowledged to be at risk include bank and building society staff, housing workers, transport staff, the police, traffic wardens, prison officers and teachers.

Violence at work is not something that should be accepted as part of the contract of employment. It cannot be dismissed as bad luck or incompetence. The nature of the work and the circumstances in which it is carried out affect the risks. Not all questions about violence will be answered but this book should help health professionals to acknowledge the risks and by doing so help them to initiate policies and procedures for the prevention and management of violence at work.

REFERENCES

D'Urso, P. and Hobbs, F.D.R. (1989) Aggression and the general practitioner. *British Medical Journal*, **298**, 97–8.
Health Services Advisory Comittee (1987) *Violence to Staff in the Health Services*, Health and Safety Commission, London.

Noble, P. and Rodger, S. (1989) Violence by psychiatric inpatients. *British Journal of Psychiatry*, **155**, 384–90.

Perkins, R. (1991) *Clinical Psychologists' Experience of Violence at Work*. Paper presented at the Annual Conference of the British Psychological Society, Bournemouth.

Rowett, C. (1986) Violence in Social Work. *Institute of Criminology Occasional Paper No. 14*, Cambridge University.

Saunders, L. (1987) *Safe and Secure in Surrey? Violence to Staff of the Social Service Department*. Social Services Research, University Department of Social Policy, Birmingham, Nos 5/6.

PART ONE

What is the risk to health care professionals?

CHAPTER 1

Violence to health care professionals: a health and safety perspective

Colin MacKay

INTRODUCTION

Violence, the subject of this book, is a topic that has received considerable attention from a wide variety of disciplines. In the context of health care the focus has been on the understanding, description and treatment of violent and aggressive patients. To the 'carers' (e.g. medical attendants, nurses and psychologists, psychiatrists) the threat of, or actual physical abuse, has been borne stoically as a truly 'occupational hazard', a matter-of-fact risk that was seen as 'part-and-parcel' of the job. For many, the caring professions are a vocation rather than a mere occupation, which probably tends to downplay feelings of threat. When incidents arose they were seen as a failure of the professional to handle difficult one-to-one situations, not a result of the need to restrain or secure severely disturbed patients. Debate was therefore focused at the **individual** level: the role of the carer, the implicit use of professional skills and the acceptable (accepted) or tolerable risks of particular tasks or jobs were presumably weighed against beneficial aspects such as self-esteem and job satisfaction.

Historically, concern about health and safety in the UK began with concern about working conditions and especially with long hours of work; an issue still of current relevance in the health service. Since then the thrust of contemporary legislation and enforcement has been directed at the elimination of hazards and reduction of risks arising from physical characteristics of the workplace. Typically these have included microbiological, chemical and radiological agents, as well as hazards from dangerous machinery. As these problems have been controlled successfully or eliminated, attention has turned to the examination of other, less recognized but no less serious, health and safety problems. One growing area of importance is the issue of violence to workers. This can be seen as a manifestation of the increasing willingness to tackle psychosocial factors in the workplace and the growing awareness of the 'human factor' in health and safety matters.

Beginning in the early 1980s, concern was being expressed by the Trade Union movement about the increasing problems of violence to staff who worked in direct contact with the public. This has led to a series of outcomes including a Committee on Violence to Staff, under the auspices of the Health and Safety Executive, a number of section specific initiatives, publications and guidance (Health Services Advisory Committee, 1987) and many local developments. While it was clear that there was a potential for violence across a range of sectors and occupational groups, progress was hampered initially by the lack of systematic data on incidence. Information was based largely upon case reports or investigations of particularly serious incidents and from more general anecdotal evidence.

THE OVERALL PICTURE

The British Crime Survey (Home Office, 1989) is an attempt to describe overall patterns of crime in the UK, including violent crimes against the person and robberies. In the 1988 British Crime Survey, a series of questions were sponsored by the Health and Safety Executive Committee on Violence, who were concerned about relative risk of particular occupational groups, with respect to actual physical assault and verbal abuse.

Earlier work in the USA and elsewhere has given a broad indication of overall patterns. First, those in paid employment are exposed to higher risks than the nonemployed (e.g. housewives, the sick, the retired) but lower than the unemployed and those still in education. Factors such as lifestyle and exposure appear to account for most of the violence. There is a five-fold greater relative risk in the most offended against than the least. Second, contextual factors also seem to have predictive value. Young, male workers in low-status, high-turnover jobs in inner city locations have the greatest risk. Third, although these demographic descriptors help to disaggregate overall patterns of risk, they give little explanation about why particular jobs are more risky. Analysis of large crime surveys, especially in the USA, highlight the following task-related factors: (i) tempting 'tools of the trade'; (ii) handling money; (iii) frequent exposure to the public; (iv) a mobile or peripatetic existence; (v) transporting goods or passengers; and (vi) work in an environment perceived to be unsafe.

Although the concern of this book is with staff in health care activities, the BCS data are helpful in providing gross comparisons of relative risk with other occupational groups. In population samples such as in the BCS, the numbers sampled in specific occupations will be usually too small to make comparisons. A condensed category has therefore been used in which 161 occupational groups are amalgamated into 17 occupational orders. Table 1.1 shows which occupational

Table 1.1 Occupations with above average job-related risks[a-c]

	Violence[d]	Threats	Thefts	Unweighted n
Education/Welfare/Health				
Higher education (men)			*	63
Teachers		**	*	172
Welfare workers	**	**		71
Medical and dental practitioners			**	22
Nurses (women)	**	**		143
Literary/artistic/sports				
All the category			*	83
Managerial[e]				
Production and site managers (men)	*			80
Officers managers (women)	**			25
Retail and wholesale managers (men)[f]	*	*	*	113
Entertainment managers	**	**	**	49
Security (men)	**	**		67
Selling				
Sales representatives (men)			*	96
Personal services				
Waitress and bar staff (women)			**	35
Houskeepers and related (women)			**	24

[a] * = at least twice average overall risk; ** = at least three times average risk. Based on incidence rates over full recall period among current workers in same job as when victimized.
[b] Categories with less than 20 workers in the sample are excluded.
[c] Weighted data. Source: 1988 BCS (core sample).
[d] 'Violence' comprises wounding, common assault and robbery; 'thefts' contact and noncontact thefts.
[e] Some nonmanagerial workers are included in security.
[f] Female retail and wholesale managers were also at risk of theft.

categories faced the highest risks and the occupational order in which they fell. Owing to the small numbers and the resultant error on the derived risk estimates, a fairly stringent criterion of vulnerability was taken. Clearly those involved in health and welfare activities figure prominently. Nevertheless these data do not help us with risks in specific jobs (e.g. ambulancemen) and ward orderlies, hospital porters and similar health care activities will be subsumed in the 'house-keeping and related' occupational group. Relative risks associated with these specific activities and jobs are discussed in the Health Services Advisory Committee (HSAC) survey. The BCS, however, gives us an overall picture of violence in this country as it relates to the workplace and to work activities. An overall summary against which the more detailed HSAC data dealing with health service staff may be compared is as follows:

1. Those who go out to work are more at risk of crime than those not in the labour force, although risks are high among the unemployed. The differences in risks among 'working women' and other women are rather less than among male workers and nonworkers – perhaps because women's lifestyles vary less whatever they do.

2. Work is the scene of much crime, although the time people spend there will largely explain this. Seven out of ten thefts of workers' personal property took place at work, although workers were not always sure who was responsible – colleagues or the public.

3. Some 14% of workers said they had been verbally abused by the public over a period of rather more than a year. Being abused becomes less frequent with age. Men and women seem equally prone.

4. Adults are most abusive. Youngsters who verbally abuse workers seem to need the company of peers more than adults, and they tend to avoid picking on men. Drunks are involved in one in ten incidents. In 80% of incidents workers were sworn at. Among non-whites, 60% of incidents involved racial abuse.

5. Workers said that one-quarter of violent offences and over one-third of the threats they experienced were the result of the work they did. A full half of threats against women were job-related but having property stolen because of their job was commoner for men.

6. Welfare workers and nurses reported comparatively high levels of violence and threats owing to their job. So too did security personnel, and those who managed places of entertainment (e.g. pubs, etc.). Teachers were not vulnerable to violence, although they were to threats, verbal abuse and thefts.

7. Offences that happened to male workers because of their jobs seemed a little more serious than other offences, although offenders were more often known. The offenders involved were older than those who caused trouble in other contexts. In 83% of violent incidents the offenders were drunk.

8. Offences that happened to women workers more often involved female young offenders, and those who were sober. Women workers reported in the rather less serious incidents in the work domain, although outside work the crimes women experienced were rather more serious than they were for men.

DESCRIBING VIOLENT INCIDENTS

Data from surveys such as the BCS provide a broad picture of categories of violent crime and estimates of relative risk in occupational groups. They thus allow the high-risk groupings to be targeted more specifically and in detail. This may be necessary because of the need to obtain a more detailed picture of the epidemiology of violent incidents in particular jobs, or because of concern about prevention and management.

Postincident narrative statements are typically unstructured and unhelpful for systematic research or data-collection purposes. Certainly, in connection with managing violence in the workplace, what is required is a practical method of investigating particular problems of violence in the particular employment situation. Anyone who has perused reports of assaults on staff knows how diverse these may be and that they can occur anywhere in a particular operation or delivery or service where staff and public interact.

As the problem of violence to staff is often associated with the main purpose of an organization the task of prevention or control can be seen to be an integral part of the management of a service or enterprise. A systematic description of the circumstances and the process are thus important and, despite the heterogeneous nature of assaults, several common themes are apparent. A simple model developed by the Tavistock Institute on behalf of HSE (Poyner and Warne, 1986, 1988) is shown in Figure 1.1. A detailed description of this model can be found in the two publications referred to, with supporting case-study material. In connection with tasks and activities carried out within a health care environment, several factors are nevertheless worth highlighting. Some aspects of health care have particular characteristics – direct physical contact is frequently involved, often in circumstances of pain or fear. This type of interaction may have been preceded by a period of waiting in a state of apprehension or uncertainty. Other factors are clearly relevant when describing the various components

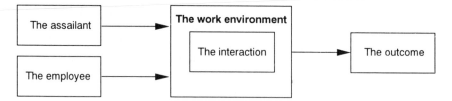

Figure 1.1 A model of violent assaults at work.

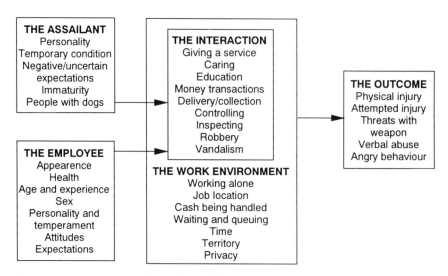

Figure 1.2 An elaborated model of violent assaults at work.

of an assault. Some of these factors, relevant to the health care environment, are shown in Figure 1.2.

EMPIRICAL EVIDENCE: THE HSAC SURVEY

In 1984, the Health Services Advisory Committee (HSAC) of the Health and Safety Commission set up a subcommittee to review the nature and size of the problem in the health service with particular reference to accident and emergency departments, community health and psychiatric care. The terms of reference of the working party specifically mentioned three areas of health care where particular problems had been identified in the past, largely through anecdotal reports, namely: accident and emergency departments, community health and psychiatric care. It was recognized that psychiatric care would represent a more complex and difficult task because of the nature of the illnesses themselves and the added dimension of long-term environmental aspects affecting staff/patient relationships and interactions.

It was also recognized that there is a potential for violence across the whole spectrum of jobs and tasks within the NHS and that, given the lack of statistical evidence on this problem, it was impossible to rule out any occupational group to whom actual violence or threat of it was insignificant. It was agreed therefore that, while particular sectors and occupations would be concentrated upon, problems inherent in other parts of the NHS would not be ignored.

In terms of incidents themselves it was felt that several fundamental questions could be posed:

1. How can violent assaults be defined and categorized?
2. What factors operate to increase or decrease the likelihood of an incident? These could be characteristics of the victim, the aggressor or the environment.
3. What jobs or occupations are most associated with risk?
4. Is violence more likely as a result of a particular activity (specificity) or is it a result of a rather nonspecific interaction?

The working party was charged with reviewing existing data on the problems of violence in the health service and, in particular, on the scale of the problems at the present time as a basis for examining the adequacy of existing policies and practices. It was clear at the outset that a major stumbling block to producing sound, reliable and workable solutions to the problem of violence was the lack of usable data on its extent in hospital and community settings.

To overcome these difficulties with existing data sources (such as they were) the working group felt it was desirable to mount an exercise of its own to obtain more reliable estimates on the size of the problem in the UK. The survey sought answers to the following questions:

1. How much violence is inflicted upon NHS staff?
2. How severe are the injuries received?
3. Are there particular groups more at risk than others?
4. The setting of the incident: are there location or time of day differences?
5. What were the contributory factors? How was the incident handled?
6. What levels and types of training have NHS staff received?

Defining what is meant by violence is an essential but difficult task for anyone involved in the investigation, management and prevention of violent incidents. For the purposes of this report and in the survey, violent incidents were classified as those:

- requiring medical assistance (major injuries): fractured bone; internal injury; unconsciousness; cut requiring stitches; deep puncture wound; hospital treatment or admission for observation;
- requiring only first aid (minor injuries): cuts, bruises, grazes; any other injury requiring treatment or requiring only 'first aid' type treatment such as a dressing or a pain killer;
- involving a threat with a weapon (no physical injury); threatened with a weapon or other object causing you to be afraid or upset even though you were not physically harmed; and
- involving verbal abuse.

Threat and verbal abuse were specifically included first because of their potential to escalate, and second, because of the serious effect of prolonged exposure to threat and verbal abuse on staff morale and efficiency.

Survey questionnaires tested in a pilot study were sent to a random sample of NHS staff working in hospitals and the community across five health authorities in different parts of the UK – including north and south, urban and rural areas. Each authority distributed 1000 questionnaires among all occupational groups, after a briefing from the working party and local consultation with managers and staff.

For those not employed directly by the health authorities, questionnaires were sent to the appropriate body for distribution following discussions and negotiations. Depending upon the area, these groups included general practitioners and their staff, ambulance staff, consultants and senior registrars.

MAIN FINDINGS OF THE HSAC SURVEY

The response rate was 60%. This figure is considered adequate for a large, mailed, self-completion survey of the sort undertaken. Response rates varied somewhat between the five areas covered and as a function of occupational group. This may reflect levels of experienced violence, attitudinal and motivational differences perhaps connected with the topic itself and ease of comprehension of the questionnaire. Large differences in experience of violence in respondents from different geographical areas were not found.

Survey respondents were predominantly female (70%) and worked full time (71%). Comparison with DHSS staffing statistics for 1985 indicated that males and full-time workers were over-represented among the respondents. They were based primarily in general hospitals (33%) and in the community setting (17%), with the remainder spread approximately equally in specialist sectors. Nearly half had been working in their present job for over 5 years (44%) and the bulk of the survey respondents had been in the health service for that time (64%).

Only 12% of those replying had received any form of training in handling violence and, of these, the majority was during basic training (76%). Of those responding to the question concerning the usefulness or otherwise of training received only 16% thought it 'extremely' useful in dealing with subsequent incidents.

INCIDENCE OF VIOLENCE

The experience of violent incidents for the survey respondents as a whole is shown in Figure 1.3. Data refer to those reporting one or more of the four categories of incident as a function of lifetime's experience, experience in current job and finally during the previous year. Analysis indicates that 1 in 200 of the respondents suffered major injury requiring medical assistance in the previous year. For the less severe categories the percentages are 11% (minor injury), 4.6% (threat with a weapon) and 17.5% (verbal threat) respectively.

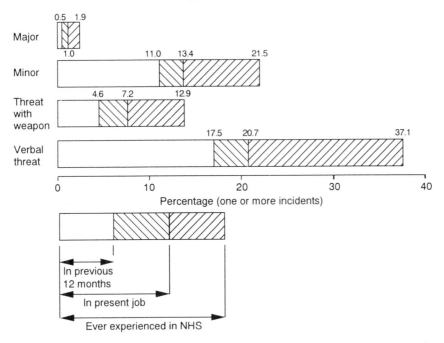

Figure 1.3 Experience of violent incidents as a function of job history and severity.

For the population as a whole comparable data are not available. A Home Office publication (Walmsley, 1986) that was published around the time of the survey gives information based on an analysis of data obtained from police forces recorded in England and Wales in 1984. Two groups of offences were considered: (i) the first, which is called 'more serious wounding', comprises attempted murder and 'wounding or other act endangering life'; (ii) the second comprised 'less serious wounding' or assault. For the more serious assaults the rates were 1 in 5300 for males and 1 in 25 000 for females. A weapon was used in about 75% of cases. For less serious wounding the rates were 1 in 310 and 1 in 880 respectively. Here a weapon was used in around 20% of cases. It must be emphasized that these figures are based upon incidents reported to the police and are therefore not strictly comparable.

Table 1.2 Reported experience of violent incidents classified by hospital type/location and by severity[a]

	Major	*Minor*	*Weapon*	*Threat*
Children's	7	92	13	138
General	2	93	46	179
Geriatric	6	213	39	152
Maternity	0	38	11	87
Mental handicap	20	209	71	199
Psychiatric	16	268	118	307
Community	2	33	39	187

[a] Data are expressed as incidence rates **per 1000** in the year immediately preceding the survey.

The incidence of violence in the previous year by overall worksite and by type of assault is shown in Table 1.2. These data support previous studies and anecdotal evidence insofar as they show high rates of more serious incidents in psychiatric facilities. Thus one in four respondents had suffered minor injury as a result of a violent attack in the year preceding the survey. Similarly high rates of assault are reportedly experienced by those working in geriatric hospitals and those in mental handicap units. Those working in maternity units and children's hospitals report least numbers of incidents overall, although those in the latter report category A (major) assaults of approaching the same frequency as colleagues in ostensibly high-risk locations. However, these rather gross comparisons mask large differences between rates within a given location. Rates for each incident type by specific location, where these data were reported by respondents for those areas showing the highest levels, are shown in Table 1.3.

Table 1.3 Experience of violent incidents by current workplace and severity[a]

	Major	Minor	Weapon	Threat
Accident and emergency	18	196	232	554
Orthopaedics	0	102	82	184
Surgical ward	0	110	96	219
Medical ward	0	262	77	385
Health centre	0	65	32	161

[a] Data expressed as incidence rates **per 1000** of those responding from the workplaces listed.

As expected, accident and emergency departments show very high rates of all assault categories, confirming earlier studies and many anecdotal reports.

A similar analysis is provided in Table 1.4 for different occupational groupings and professional categories. Data are categorized by current job title by incident type in the previous year (i.e. the last 12 months). Since fine distinctions between job titles have been drawn, the numbers in some occupational groups are quite low – especially for category A (major) injuries – and absolute frequencies are sometimes very small. Their use as true estimates of actual risk must therefore be treated with caution. Again these data confirm previous suggestions as to the high risk of some groups working in the community especially ambulancemen and certain nursing grades.

Table 1.4 Reported incidence of violent incidents classified by some selected occupational groups and by severity[a]

	Major	Minor	Weapon	Threat
Hospital doctors	5	59	30	193
GPs	5	5	50	249
Student nurse	16	364	136	402
Staff nurse	0	202	73	337
Charge nurse	16	172	86	242
Ambulance staff	17	174	174	421
Catering	0	11	11	11
Laundry	0	20	0	59
Domestic	6	30	30	42
Porters	0	81	32	210

[a] Data are expressed as incidence rates **per 1000** in the year preceding the survey.

Approximate estimates of patient contact were derived from respondents (five categories ranging from 0–10% to 76–100%).

Table 1.5 Percentage of respondents reporting one or more incidents as a function of patient contact and type of incident in the previous 12 months

Incident category	*Proportion of working time spent dealing with patients/relatives*				
	0–10%	*10–25%*	*25–50%*	*50–75%*	*75–100%*
Major	0	0	0.9	0.6	0.7
Minor	2.4	7.4	13.7	11.9	16.3
Weapon	1.4	3.0	6.4	4.1	7.1
Threat	3.9	14.5	21.1	22.4	24.8

Table 1.5 shows the percentage of respondents reporting one or more incidents in the last 12 months as a function of patient contact and type of incident. Overall the relative risk of assault is in the order of 1:6 between the lowest and highest level of exposure irrespective of incident type.

THE INCIDENTS THEMSELVES

There was little overall evidence of assaults being more prevalent on particular days of the week. The only clearly elevated risk appeared to be on Fridays so far as major injuries were concerned; this accounted for 26% of all cases. Similarly, there was little evidence of large time-of-day differences in the likelihood of assault. Overall the level of assaults was highest in the busiest part of the day (lunchtime, afternoon) and lowest in the early hours of the morning (03.00–09.00 h). The assailant was, in most cases, a patient or client irrespective of incident type (85% major injury, 75% verbal threat). In the remainder of cases, the assailant was a relative or friend of the patient. There was some evidence that the more serious incidents were characterized by a lack of warning of an impending assault and victims were more often alone compared with less serious incidents. In cases of assaults involving major injury, 30% involved a weapon, one in ten of victims were admitted to hospital and 37% subsquently had more than 3 days sickness absence. In the case of minor injury, only 1% of the cases had greater than 3 days absence. Detailed analysis by specific workplace indicated that some locations had proportionately higher levels of violence than others. As expected, those working in accident and emergency departments reported the highest levels.

Irrespective of severity of incident one-third of those responding said there was an agreed procedure to follow in the circumstances in which they found themselves. Official recording of the incident took place in 70% of cases of major injury. For minor injury, threat with a weapon and verbal threat the figures were 35%, 31% and 18% respectively.

CONCLUSIONS

Based upon the results of the present survey, violence towards staff, whether causing actual bodily harm or being psychologically threatening or stressful, is a significant problem. The problem is not narrowly concentrated but seems to afflict a range of occupations, in a range of activities both in the hospital setting and the community. There are, however, some high-risk settings that have been identified by the survey and which confirm previously held views. Ambulance staff, nurses (particularly the training grades), accident and emergency departments and caring for psychologically disturbed individuals reported the highest level of risk.

Overall, the survey results pointed towards several factors associated with the likelihood of attack but three of these – training, working practices and procedural issues – seemed particularly salient.

Violence has implications both for the health authority as an organization and also for the individual at risk. For the organization it is disruptive, impairs organizational effectiveness and may be costly in terms of staff morale and efficiency as well as in lost time through sickness absence.

For the individual at risk there is the worry and anxiety caused by the probability of likely assault, as well as the undesirable consequences of actual physical attack. That violence is a complex topic is illustrated by the data from the present survey as well as from previous studies. Many interacting factors are involved in determining whether a particular situation or event will escalate into a violent attack. As well as those highlighted above, some of the more important ones are: (i) the potential aggressor – his or her present medical and psychological state and known history of violence; (ii) the victim – coping and interpersonal skills and physical size; (iii) the nature of the interaction between these two people at the time and what activities were underway; and (iv) their individual perception of threat of each other or the situation and the physical setting or environment. All of these factors are likely to be important and are more or less amenable to change or manipulation by way of prevention and management.

A systematic approach to the problem of violence is essential if the policies for dealing with the risk are to be effective. The general guidance set out in HSE publications (Poyner and Warne, 1986, 1988) together with the more specific guidance covering the health service (Health Services Advisory Committee, 1987; Department of Health and Social Security, 1988) are designed to help with developing a coherent approach to prevention and management. The issue of violence is likely to be of growing concern in the next decade. This book will help to refocus attention on this important topic, which in turn should help to safeguard the health, safety and well-being of staff who are striving to deliver a high-quality service to their patients and customers.

REFERENCES

Department of Health and Social Security (1988) *Violence to Staff. Report of the DHSS Advisory Committee on Violence to Staff*. HMSO, London.

Health Services Advisory Committee (1987) *Violence to Staff in the Health Services*, HMSO, London.

Home Office Research and Planning Unit (Mayhew, P., Elliot, D. and Dowds, L.) (1989) *The 1988 British Crime Survey*. HMSO, London.

Poyner, B. and Warne, C. (1986) *Violence to Staff – A Basis for Assessment and Prevention*. Health and Safety Executive. HMSO, London.

Poyner, B. and Warne, C. (1988) *Preventing Violence to Staff*. Health and Safety Executive. HMSO, Lonodn.

Walmsley, R. (1986) *Personal Violence*. Home Office Research Study No. 89. Home Office Research and Planning Unit, HMSO, London.

CHAPTER 2

Violence in psychiatric hospitals

Richard Whittington

INTRODUCTION

Violence was recognized and acknowledged as a problem in psychiatric hospitals much sooner than in other settings and, as a result, more research has been carried out in hospitals. In this chapter three main aspects of violence in psychiatric hospitals will be discussed: (i) the nature of such violence (frequency and severity); (ii) the patients who are more likely to engage in such behaviour; and (iii) the situations where violence is more likely to occur. It will become clear that recent research has focused on the first two areas and insufficient attention has been paid to the assaultive situation. Only when environmental and interpersonal factors are included in our explanations of why violence occurs in psychiatric hospitals will effective interventions to deal with the problem be made.

It is apparent that violence in psychiatric hospitals has been recognized as a problem since at least the latter part of the 19th century. For instance, Ekblom (1970) briefly describes three studies by German psychiatrists conducted in the 1880s and 1890s. Although the problem was acknowledged very early, however, there was little research interest before 1970. In contrast, the past 20 years has witnessed a vast increase in the number of publications on the problem. This proliferation started in America in the 1970s with the work of clinicians such as John Lion (e.g. Lion and Reid, 1983) and Kenneth Tardiff (e.g. Tardiff and Sweillam, 1982) but interest has now spread to the UK. Interest in violence by clinicians has been paralleled by a growing willingness amongst government and other agencies to consider the problem (DHSS, 1976, 1986, 1988; Health Services Advisory Committee, 1987; Poyner and Warne, 1986).

It has been claimed that this contemporary concern among staff and employers is a response to increased levels of violence in society in general, and health care settings in particular. Home Office research (Walmsley, 1986) has documented how offences of violence against the person increased by 52% between 1974 and 1984 and a recent review of violence in psychiatric hospitals included the claim that:

> Considerable evidence has been marshalled .. to indicate that assaults on staff have increased substantially over the past 10 years.
>
> (*Haller and Deluty, 1988*)

Indeed, several British studies have shown an increase in rates of violence from one year to the next (e.g. Hodgkinson *et al.*, 1985; James *et al.*, 1990) and data from a large, longitudinal study of several thousand incidents over 13 years (Noble and Rodger, 1989) demonstrated that the average number of violent incidents reported per year in the 1980s was nearly three times that reported in the latter part of the 1970s.

However, some of these claims must be treated with caution. Haller and Deluty's (1988) evidence for an increase in violence, evidence that they regard as 'considerable', amounts to one study in a mid-Western American private hospital (Adler *et al.*, 1983) and a personal communication to the authors. That studies show a year-on-year increase is also of limited value since such an increase may equally be due to sensitization among staff.

What is likely to have changed in the past 20 years in addition to increased rates of violence is **tolerance** of such assaultive behaviour by patients. For many years, violence to staff in psychiatric hospitals was probably seen as 'part of the job', an unpleasant experience but an unavoidable occupational hazard. Now it is possible that both staff and their employers are beginning to consider violence by patients as unacceptable behaviour because of the serious consequences for all those involved.

In this context it is interesting to compare 'old' and 'new' definitions of aggression. A study by the German psychiatrist Laehr carried out in 1889 (cited by Ekblom, 1970) concerned itself exclusively with the murder of psychiatrists. In contrast, modern studies of violence at work tend to include verbal abuse and threats (to all staff) in their definitions of aggressive behaviour (Health Services Advisory Committee, 1987), and some include sexual harassment or indeed any behaviour perceived by the victim to be hostile (Saunders, 1991). It is clear that the boundaries of what is and what is not acceptable behaviour by psychiatric patients in hospital have shifted markedly over the past century and most quickly over the past 20 years.

It is not immediately apparent why such a shift in tolerance should have taken place. Some relevant factors may be increased self-respect and status among staff working in psychiatric settings, concern among trade unions (COHSE, 1976) and a recent concern in society with the experience of victims. An important influence is likely to have been the recognition by managers and the government that violence to their staff is a problem not only for which they have responsibility under the Health and Safety at Work Act but which can also cost them significant amounts of money. The chairperson of the Health and Safety Commission has written that:

> Working in an atmosphere of continuing threat is profoundly damaging to the confidence and morale of staff. For employers, there are costs in terms of reduced efficiency, sickness absence, and a bad 'image', inhibiting future recruitment.
>
> *(Cullen in HSAC, 1987)*

In America, Lanza and Milner (1989) attempted to estimate exactly how much of a drain on resources violence to staff in psychiatric hospitals might be. In an article entitled '*The dollar cost of patient assault*', they estimated the cost of each assault by investigating a wide variety of organizational procedures that have to be implemented as a result of each assault. These procedures included such things as administrative time dealing with paperwork, counselling and support for victims, safety issues and training for staff. When all this had been computed, Lanza and Milner (1989) estimated that the average assault on staff in an American psychiatric hospital costs about $575 (about £300 at the present exchange rate). If these data are applied to the British health service, where one in ten of the 1 000 000 employees receives physical injury from an assault every year (Health Services Advisory Committee, 1987), violence to health care professionals may cost the government here as much as £30 000 000 a year. Violence to NHS staff in general, and staff in psychiatric hospitals in particular, is therefore a significant problem.

THE NATURE OF VIOLENCE IN PSYCHIATRIC SETTINGS

Although an extensive research effort has been made to deal with this problem in the USA (Davis, 1991, for a review), the emphasis here will be on UK research because transatlantic comparisons on rates of violence are difficult to draw. American society is known to be more aggressive than that in Britain (Walmsley, 1986) and there is evidence that violence is more common and severe in American psychiatric settings. Edwards *et al.* (1988) have estimated that the violence rate in the psychiatric unit of a District General Hospital (DGH) in Southampton was about one-quarter of that occurring in US psychiatric hospitals. In addition, violence in US psychiatric settings may be more physically severe than that occurring in the UK. While 73% of nurses assaulted in Ryan and Poster's (1989) study suffered physical injury, only about 40% of assaults in UK psychiatric settings lead to such injuries (Noble and Rodger, 1989). As a result of these factors, there is a different set of attitudes in America to the problem of violence and some of these attitudes may shock UK professionals. This is most eloquently revealed by the routine recommendation of an American nurse that 'security personnel **must remove their guns before entering** an inpatient unit' (Kronberg, 1983).

Modern research into violence in British psychiatric hospitals began with Fottrell's (1980) survey comparing rates of violence in one urban and one rural psychiatric hospital with those in a District General Hospital psychiatric unit. A flood of studies then followed, with 11 surveys of violence in British psychiatric hospitals and units published between 1982 and 1990. Some aspects of these surveys are summarized in Table 2.1.

There are problems in comparing the results of the 12 studies because each approaches the problem in slightly different ways. The settings of each study must be borne in mind since violence in a Special Hospital (e.g. Rampton) is markedly different from that occurring in the psychiatric unit of a District General Hospital. More importantly, many studies rely on official report forms for their sample of violent incidents. This is a notoriously unreliable system for getting an accurate picture of the real problem of violence (Archer, 1989) since up to four out of every five incidents are not reported (Lion *et al.*, 1981). Other problems with relying on official report forms are the deterioration of memory for events over a period of hours, the fact that staff who did not witness the incident may complete the form and the motivation of participants to describe events truthfully.

A third problem with comparisons between studies listed in Table 2.1 is that the type of violence under investigation varies between them. Most of the studies clearly state that they are concerned with physical violence but a few are not explicit and may include verbal assault (threats, abuse) in their remit. More importantly, while all the studies examined assaults on staff, some of them included assaults on other patients, violence to property and even self-harm in their sample, so they are not all discussing the same type of event.

Target of violence

The concern of this chapter is assaults on staff, and it is necessary to examine how often violence to staff occurs compared with the other types of violence. A basic distinction in definitions of aggressive behaviour is whether such aggression is directed inwards (i.e. self-harm) or outwards. When self-harm is included in the definition

Table 2.1 Studies of violence in British and Eire psychiatric hospitals 1980–1990

Study	Setting	Detection of incidents	Type of violence				
			To staff	To patients	To self	To property	Threats
Fottrell (1980)	Two hospitals and one DGH unit	'Reliable reporting'	Yes	Yes	Yes	No	No
Armond (1982)	Semi-secure ward	Doctor on the ward, nursing and medical notes reviewed	Yes	Yes	No	Yes	No
Drinkwater (1982)	Three wards	Participant observation	Yes	Yes	Yes	Yes	No
Cooper et al. (1983)	Female observation ward	Senior nurse on duty completed form	Yes	Yes	?	?	?
Aiken (1984)	Locked ward	Incident form, ?doctor on ward	Yes	No	No	No	No
Hodgkinson et al. (1985)	Psychiatric hospital	Incident reports	Yes	No	No	No	No
Convey (1986)	Acute admission ward	Incident reports, ?nurse on ward	Yes	Yes	No	Yes	No
Pearson et al. (1986)	Psychiatric hospital	Incident reports	Yes	Yes	No	Yes	No
Dooley (1986)	Forensic hospital (Eire)	Incident reports	Yes	Yes	Yes	Yes	No
Edwards et al. (1988)	DGH psychiatric unit	Ward contacted three times/week	Yes	Yes	No	No	No
Larkin et al. (1988)	Special hospital	Weekly visits to ward	Yes	Yes	Yes	Yes	No
Noble and Rodger (1989)	Two psychiatric hospitals	Incident reports	Yes	Yes	No	Yes	No
James et al. (1990)	High-dependency ward	Incident reports	Yes	Yes	Yes	Yes	No

of aggression, it is relatively uncommon compared with violence directed outwards (e.g. Cooper *et al.*, 1983). Dooley's (1986) survey of an Irish Special Hospital is unusual in finding self-harm more frequent than violence to staff or property and this may reflect the special conditions applying in a forensic hospital.

A further distinction can also be made between violence to inanimate objects, such as furniture, and that directed toward people (interpersonal violence). Violence to property is also usually less common than interpersonal assaults (James *et al.*, 1990), although it seems likely that staff are more likely to report interpersonal violence than property violence since such aggression may be seen as having more serious consequences.

Finally, it may be important to distinguish between violence to other patients and violence to staff. Haller and Deluty (1988) propose that the dynamics of the two types of assault are different. Violence to other patients may be influenced by ward hierarchies and take place when violence to staff is not seen as an option (Depp, 1983). However, there is little consistency between the studies over whether interpersonal violence is directed more often at staff or other patients. Most studies report that staff are assaulted more often than patients (Noble and Rodger, 1989) but the differences are often small.

One very clear message from the studies of violence in hospital, regardless of their various methods of tackling the problem, is that, when assaults on staff are considered in isolation, there is a consistent trend for nurses to be assaulted more frequently than other staff groups. Table 2.2 illustrates that every study that provides a breakdown of assaults according to occupational group reports that most assaults are directed against nurses, and all but one of the studies estimate that the proportion is about 90%. Similar proportions have been reported in the USA (Carmel and Hunter, 1989). This is not likely to be due merely to the large numbers of nurses in the workforce of psychiatric hospitals and units because in an unpublished victimization survey by Roscoe (1987) nurses made up only 48% of the workforce of a psychiatric hospital, while experiencing 83% of assaults on staff.

Table 2.2 Proportion of assaults on staff directed against nurses

Study	Number of assaults on staff (n)	Percentage directed against nurses (%)
Armond (1982)	17	88.2
Cooper *et al.* (1983)	92	95.6
Aiken (1984)	41	90.2
Hodgkinson *et al.* (1985)	622	94.0
Edwards *et al.* (1988)	23	65.2
Larkin *et al.* (1988)	407	90.9
Noble and Rodger (1989)	89	87.6

Different grades of nursing staff are assaulted at widely differing rates but there is little agreement over which grades face most risk of assault. Hodgkinson *et al.* (1985) report that **student nurses** were significantly more likely to be assaulted than would be expected from their numbers in the workforce; they suggest that this might be because they are relatively inexperienced and regularly change wards, which prevents them establishing relationships with patients. The permanence of staff and their consequent ability to get to know patients seems to be important because James *et al.* (1990) found that the rate of violent incidents increased as the number of shifts worked by **agency staff** increased. However Convey (1986) found over one-third of assaults were made on the two **nursing assistants** on her ward (10% of the staff), which she suggests may be because they spend longer with patients than other grades, they are untrained and they may be unsure of treatment decisions as they rarely participate in ward conferences.

Of course, nurses are not the only staff group to be assaulted by patients. Other staff groups specified as being assaulted include doctors (Aiken, 1984; Noble and Rodger, 1989), occupational therapists (Larkin *et al.*, 1988) and domestic staff (Hodgkinson *et al.*, 1985) but these groups are known to be assaulted less often than might be expected from their presence in the workforce (Roscoe, 1987).

Frequency of assaults on staff

It is possible to make a rough estimate of how often staff in psychiatric settings are likely to experience violence by combining the information from the 12 British and Eire studies (see Table 2.3).

It is clear from Table 2.3 that rates of assault vary widely from one study to the next. While in one Special Hospital an assault was reported less than once a fortnight, in the other an assault was reported on average every 10 hours. When individual wards and units are compared, there is similar variation. The semi-secure ward investigated by Armond (1982) had less than one assault every month, while the female observation unit examined by Cooper *et al.* (1983) had an assault every other day. Local factors other than the location and type of unit must be relevant in determining the levels of violence experienced in each of these settings. These factors will include patient characteristics and situational aspects.

Nevertheless, despite the variation, it is possible to draw some conclusions about the frequency of assaults on staff. The average rate for **hospitals** is one assault every 6 days and that for **individual units** is one assault every 11 days. The average in urban hospitals is higher than that in rural hospitals and that in specialist units is higher than that in general units and hospitals overall. This is not surprising since rates of violence are usually higher in urban areas than rural areas and disturbed patients cared for on specialist units are more likely to engage in violent behaviour (Lowenstein *et al.*, 1990). However, the main conclusion must be that the **average** frequency of assaults on staff in psychiatric hospitals is every 11 days. Obviously some units will experience assaults at a higher rate than this and many other units will pass through phases when they exceed the average number of assaults. Therefore violent victimization of oneself or colleagues is far from being a rare event in the working lives of staff in psychiatric hospitals. Although most assaults will result in no significant physical injury, the cumulative effect of being exposed to regular violence may be one way in which such an event becomes a significant occupational stressor for staff.

Table 2.3 Rate of assaults on staff in British and Eire psychiatric hospitals

Study	Number of assaults on staff	Length of study (days)	Days per assault
HOSPITALS			
(a) Urban			
Fottrell (1980)	243	365	1.5
Hodgkinson *et al.* (1985)	622	720	1.2
(b) Rural			
Fottrell (1980)	25	365	14.6
Pearson *et al.* (1986)	92	365	4.0
(c) Special			
Dooley (1986)	20	365	18.2
Larkin *et al.* (1988)	407	180	0.4
UNITS			
(a) Specialist			
Armond (1982)	17	630	37.0
Cooper *et al.* (1983)	88	180	2.0
Aiken (1984)	41	180	4.4
James *et al.* (1990)	44	450	10.2
(b) General			
Fottrell (1980)	17	120	7.0
Convey (1986)	32	180	5.6
Edwards *et al.* (1988)	23	365	15.8

Severity of assaults

The severity of an assault can be measured in two ways. Most of the studies provide information on the physical consequences of the assault and use this to assess the severity of the event. This approach was first used by Fottrell (1980) and his classification system is still widely used, both in the UK and the USA:

• Grade 1 No physical injury detectable or suspected;

- Grade 2 Minor physical injuries, e.g. bruises, abrasions, small lacerations; and
- Grade 3 Major physical injury (e.g. large lacerations, fractures, loss of consciousness); need for special investigations (e.g. blood test) irrespective of findings; permanent physical disability or death.

Studies that use this classification have found that the majority of assaults result in no detectable or suspected injury. A smaller proportion result in grade 2 injuries and a tiny proportion result in major physical injury. The largest survey, of more than 12 000 assaults over 13 years (Noble and Rodger, 1989), found that 59% of incidents were grade 1, 39% grade 2 and 2% grade 3. Several studies with relatively large samples found the proportion of assaults resulting in major injuries to be under 1% (e.g. Pearson *et al.*, 1986). There is also evidence that assaults on staff are less physically severe than those made against patients (Pearson *et al.*, 1986). Again, it should be noted that the situation may be different in Special Hospitals as Larkin *et al.* (1988) report that nearly half the assaults at Rampton resulted in minor injury and 10 assaults on nurses were life-threatening (in 6 months). Drinkwater (1982) considered the severity of assaults in a different way and examined the nature of the violence that took place. She reports that over half the assaults (63%) included punching, 47% pushing, 33% kicking, 27% scratching and 26% slapping of the victim.

There is growing evidence, however, that the severity of assaults cannot be only considered in terms of the physical injury suffered by the victim. It seems likely that victims will experience some psychological trauma following assaults, regardless of the physical injury they sustain (see Chapter 6). A growing number of studies have demonstrated such effects (Lanza, 1983; Ryan and Poster, 1989) and sometimes significant psychological distress occurs in the absence of significant physical injury (Whittington and Wykes, 1992). The factors that influence such stress reactions are not yet clear but may be caused by the appraisal of threat in an incident and repeated exposure to the 'daily hassle' of so-called 'minor' assaults (Lazarus and Folkman, 1984).

Summary

This section has been concerned with the 'epidemiology' of violence in psychiatric hospitals. The main conclusions are:

- that most assaults on staff are directed against nurses and that this is not simply due to their greater numbers in the workforce;
- that assaults on staff take place on average between every 6 and 11 days;
- that few assaults result in significant physical injury; but

- that even assaults that do not result in such injury may still result in severe psychological distress for the victim.

THE ASSAULTIVE PATIENT

Having gained some understanding of the nature of violence in psychiatric hospitals, the next step is to identify why such behaviour occurs. It may be due to the types of individual who are cared for within such settings ('person' factors) and there is some evidence (reviewed by Howells, 1982) that, in general, mentally disordered people are more likely to engage in violent behaviour than other people. Conversely, the aggression in psychiatric hospitals may be due to aspects of the hospital environment or routine that are unpleasant enough to make anybody aggressive, regardless of mental illness or other individual factors. Being forced to stay in the hospital is an example of such a 'situational' factor. Most of the research into violence in psychiatric hospitals has examined the 'person' factors, especially mental illness, thus it is possible to present a relatively detailed picture of the violent psychiatric patient. Much less effort has been made to investigate the 'situation' factors that contribute to violent behaviour in psychiatric hospitals but an attempt will be made in the next section to outline what is known and to draw some conclusions. Undoubtedly, it will not be possible to understand fully and deal with violence to staff unless both 'person' and 'situation' factors are included in the explanation.

A reasonably consistent picture of the 'assaultive patient' has emerged from the studies under discussion. One consistent and reassuring finding is that only a minority of psychiatric patients act aggressively and most studies estimate that something between one-quarter and one-third of general psychiatric patients in hospital behave aggressively during their admission (e.g. Pearson *et al.*, 1986). Not only is it usually a minority of patients who are ever aggressive, it is also a small minority of **that** minority who are aggressive repeatedly. Less than half the aggressive patients were violent more than once in most studies and a small group of patients often featured in a greatly disproportionate number of assaults. Hodgkinson *et al.* (1985), for instance, report that 12 patients (1.4% of the hospital population and 5% of the aggressive population) were involved in one-quarter of all assaults in the hospital. One patient in the study by Larkin *et al.* (1988) of 154 aggressive patients accounted for 12% of assaults.

Clinical features

The mental illness of the patient is likely to be an important factor in explaining violence in psychiatric hospitals. The diagnosis of the patient is a useful predictor of violence risk since it has been found that schizophrenic patients present a significantly greater risk of aggressive behaviour than patients with other diagnoses (e.g. Noble and Rodger, 1989). Armond (1982) found that half the assaults in his study involved three patients with schizophrenia (out of 40 patients in all) and Aiken (1984) also found that the four most frequently assaultative patients had a diagnosis of schizophrenia. The risk presented by patients from other diagnostic groups is not so clear, although several studies report a high involvement of patients with manic-depressive disorder in assaults (e.g. James *et al.*, 1990). Conversely, those who are neurotic or depressed, have a dementing illness and those with personality and addictive disorders have all been found to present a **reduced** risk in some studies.

There are limits, however, to the usefulness of a diagnosis for explaining the occurrence of aggressive behaviour since patients may not be symptomatic at the time of the assault. Aggression by a schizophrenic patient, for instance, may be the result of psychopathology associated with their illness but it may also be due to other factors such as personality. It is desirable therefore to obtain more up-to-date information on specific psychopathology at the time of the violence. When this has been attempted, it is clear that the key symptoms with regard to aggressive behaviour are **delusions** and **hallucinations** (Cooper *et al.*, 1983; Aiken, 1984; Sheridan *et al.*, 1990; see also the studies reviewed in Chapter 6). Noble and Rodger (1989), for instance, found that violent patients were significantly more likely to be hallucinated and deluded than other patients, thus implicating active psychosis in the occurrence of aggression. Patients themselves sometimes also acknowledge the importance of hallucinations in causing their own aggressive behaviour (Cooper *et al.*, 1983). Other aspects of mental disorder that may be relevant to aggressive behaviour are **drug or alcohol intoxication** and **confusion** due to a dementing illness (Sheridan *et al.*, 1990).

It is important to specify how these disorders may contribute to the occurrence of aggressive behaviour. Confusion, intoxication and psychosis are similar in that they impair the person's ability to interpret accurately the behaviour of other people. Geen (1990) emphasizes the importance of judgements or **appraisal** of a situation as a determinant of angry feelings and aggressive behaviour. If, for instance, a patient is frustrated by a member of staff, the patient is more likely to feel angry and aggressive toward the staff member if their actions seem 'arbitrary, malicious or intentional' (p. 51). Alternatively, if the frustration appears in some ways 'justifiable or normal', relatively little anger will be experienced. Confused or intoxicated patients may be particularly prone to appraising staff behaviour as arbitrary since they do not understand the reasons why the staff are behaving in a particular way. Paranoid or deluded patients are likely to interpret staff behaviour as intentionally malicious towards them. Some experiments have shown how deluded patients often interpret the emotions communicated by facial expressions differently from the interpretations made by nondeluded people (Cutting, 1981; Walker *et al.*, 1984) so that a friendly expression may be misinterpreted as hostile. Thus patients experiencing these symptoms appraise staff behaviour in a way that makes them more likely to experience arousal and anger leading to aggression.

Other factors

Many other aspects of violent patients have been investigated in an attempt to identify those who present an increased risk to staff. Demographic characteristics are of limited use in identifying potentially aggressive psychiatric inpatients. The most useful demographic predictor is the **age** of the patient since it is well known that younger patients seem to present a higher risk than other age groups. Several studies (e.g. Noble and Rodger, 1989) have found that patients either in their late teens or twenties were involved in significantly more assaults than might be expected. However, it is not recognized so widely that older patients may also present a significant risk. Both Noble and Rodger (1989) and Hodgkinson *et al.* (1985) found that patients in their seventies were involved in a disproportionate number of assaults. Staff should be aware, as warned by Noble and Rodger (1989), that some aggression occurs throughout the age range and should not underestimate the risks of working with older patients. In a survey of staff working with geriatric patients (Health Services Advisory Committee, 1987), over one-fifth had received physical injury from assault by a patient over 12 months (see also Colenda and Hamer, 1991).

With regard to **gender**, since physical violence by males in society is far more common than such behaviour by females (Walmsley, 1986) it might be anticipated that male patients present more of a risk to staff than females; however, this is not necessarily the case. Hodgkinson *et al.* (1985) found no difference in the frequencies with which males and females were involved in violence and Larkin *et al.* (1988) actually found females involved more often than males. Females below or in their twenties may present a particular risk to staff (Hodgkinson *et al.*, 1985; Convey, 1986). As Convey points out, this may be because staff are more willing to confront female patients on their own and thus place themselves at more risk than if the patient was male. The same underestimation of danger may apply to the care of older patients. Another aspect of the gender difference is that men and women may be violent in different ways. Noble and Rodger (1989) note that all three grade 3 incidents in their study involved males and that each gender used different types of weapon. Armond (1982) also notes that males tended to assault with their fists while females threw objects.

Other demographic characteristics such as **ethnic origin** and **social situation** have been studied and no relationship with aggressive behaviour was apparent (James *et al.*, 1990; Noble and Rodger, 1989).

Since, as we have seen, many violent patients are repeatedly aggressive, their **history of violence** should be useful in establishing the risk. It is surprising that relatively little UK research attention has been paid to this factor but those studies that have examined history of violence support its validity as a predictor. Aiken (1984) reports that all but one of the 19 aggressive patients in his study had a history of previous violence and Noble and Rodger (1989) report that aggressive patients were significantly more likely to have previously damaged property or been verbally aggressive and threatening. In Norway, Blomhoff *et al.* (1990) found that history of previous violence alone correctly identified 80% of patients who were violent following admission to hospital (Chapter 6).

With regard to **legal status**, it is also not surprising that violent patients are often detained compulsorily since presenting a danger to other people is often a criterion for 'sectioning'. James *et al.* (1990) found that violent patients were significantly more likely to have been admitted compulsorily compared with nonviolent patients, while Noble and Rodger (1989) found that violent patients were significantly more likely than nonviolent patients to have been sectioned at some point **during** the admission. Legal detention often took place as a result of violence within the hospital. However, it is important to note that violence may result from sectioning as well as being a cause of such action. The potential for aggressive behaviour ('fight') is increased when escape from an unpleasant situation ('flight') is not permissible (Owens and Bagshaw, 1985) so that patients forced to stay in such situations are more likely to become aggressive. In addition, many assaults on staff occur directly as a result of preventing patients from leaving the ward on which they are detained.

A wide variety of other factors that may identify potentially violent patients have been studied in the USA. For example, Convit *et al.* (1988) report the development of a 'risk-factor profile' where the presence of a combination of neurological abnormalities (e.g. abnormal EEG), histories of violent crime and violent suicide attempts and also deviant family environments in childhood, were found to predict accurately whether particular patients would be aggressive in hospital. While this research is promising, at the moment it is of limited practical use to health care professionals who may have no access to such detailed information.

Summary

Most research into violence in psychiatric hospitals attempts to identify the characteristics of 'the violent patient' and certain conclusions can be drawn:

- only a minority of psychiatric patients engage in aggressive behaviour and only a small proportion are aggressive repeatedly;
- patients who are (i) under 30 years of age, (ii) diagnosed as having schizophrenia (especially if actively psychotic), (iii) detained under the Mental Health Act, or (iv) known to have a history of previous violence, present particularly high risks of aggression to staff; and
- the risks of violence by older patients and female patients should not be underestimated by staff.

THE ASSAULTIVE SITUATION

To complement this picture of 'the violent patient' it is necessary to examine some of the situational factors that may contribute to violence occurring in psychiatric hospitals. Much of the research into violence in psychiatric hospitals is based on what might be called a 'radically individualistic' perspective (Depp, 1983), whereby violence by psychiatric patients is viewed as virtually 'the spontaneous manifestation of underlying psychopathology' (Davis, 1991). Yet psychological theories of aggression specify a wide variety of inter-personal and environmental factors that make aggression by humans (whether mentally ill or not) more likely to occur. Interpersonal factors such as the behaviour of other people, in this case staff or other patients, are well established as important precursors of violence yet have been relatively ignored in previous research.

Timing and location of assaults

Circumstantial evidence for the importance of situational influences comes from the apparent 'ebb and flow' of violence over time. Peaks of violence seem to occur on particular weekdays in different units (Larkin *et al.*, 1988; Cooper *et al.*, 1983). These weekdays vary according to the individual unit being studied and are presumed to reflect the particular events occurring on the wards on these days, for example a ward round. Peaks have also been reported in the morning (Hodgkinson *et al.*, 1985) and at mealtimes (Pearson *et al.*, 1986). In contrast, rates of violence tend to ebb at weekends and during the night (Noble and Rodger, 1989).

In terms of location of aggression, admission wards are consistently reported to suffer high levels of violence (Larkin *et al.*, 1988), which presumably reflects the relatively unstable nature of staff–patient relationships within such units. The early part of an admission may be particularly difficult (Convey, 1986) since disturbance may be at its highest and security has not been established. There is no consistency over the rates of violence experienced by different types of unit and this may well reflect their particular cultures. Secure wards, psycho-geriatric wards and drug dependency units have all been found to have low rates of aggression in some studies (e.g. Pearson *et al.*, 1986) and high rates in others (e.g. Fottrell, 1980). Within the ward, certain areas may be the site of more assaults than others, for instance the dining room (Cooper *et al.*, 1983) or entrance/exit to the unit (Convey, 1986).

Antecedents of assaults

More direct evidence for the importance of interpersonal and situational factors comes from studies that attempt to identify the precursors of violent incidents. Drinkwater (1982) emphasizes the importance of the nature of interaction, particularly staff–patient interaction, occurring on psychiatric wards as an influence on violent behaviour. Two types of antecedent event seem to be of particular importance. First, there are occasions when patients are angered or annoyed by the intrusive or frustrating behaviour of other people. This 'aversive stimulation' may come from other patients on the ward (Cooper *et al.*, 1983; Sheridan *et al.*, 1990), for example, when there are disputes over cigarettes or food (Aiken, 1984) or it may result from the behaviour of staff themselves. It is often inherent in the task of 'caring' for psychiatric patients that staff have to intrude upon or frustrate the patient and this is a common precursor of violence. Several different antecedent events have been described, such as preventing the patient from leaving the ward (Convey, 1986), disputes over medication (Aiken, 1984) and general enforcement of rules or denial of requests (Sheridan *et al.*, 1990). Information from a Canadian study by Cooper and Medonca (1991) indicates that some of these ante-cedents consist of physical behaviour (e.g. restraining, physically guiding or leading, taking something from or lifting the patient) while others are merely verbal statements (requesting the patient to do or stop doing something). Such intrusive or frustrating behaviour, however well-meaning by staff, has been established clearly as a significant contributor to aggressive behaviour in humans, although the likelihood of aggression may be reduced by influencing the patient's appraisal of the interaction. Thus the staff behaviour should be explained and justified to the patient whenever possible to avoid appraisal of the situation as arbitrary or malicious.

It should also be noted that the person who is assaulted may not be the person who angered or annoyed the patient since aggression can often be displaced onto more accessible targets. Thus staff may be assaulted because of provocations by other patients since staff may be perceived as unable to retaliate because of their professional role. Alternatively, other patients may be assaulted when staff have angered a patient since staff are seen as a more powerful and dangerous adversary (Depp, 1983).

The second type of antecedent that may be relevant to violence in psychiatric hospitals is the opposite to that just described. Rather than objecting to the intrusive nature of enforced interaction with other people, it has been suggested that some patients find being left on their own aversive and therefore become aggressive in order to force staff to interact with them. Drinkwater (1982) argues that more disturbed patients are avoided by staff because interaction with them is found to be difficult and stressful. These patients are put in the position where they have to use 'extreme behaviour such as violence' to gain staff attention. Thus staff 'reward' this antisocial behaviour by interacting with the patient only at the times of acting violently and therefore make it more likely to occur again. There is some support for the idea that some patients find lack of staff attention an aversive situation that they can remedy by becoming violent because in one study one-quarter of violent incidents were seen as 'attention-seeking behaviour' by staff (Cooper *et al.*, 1983).

It is sometimes the case that, rather than particular individual patients being ostracized, all the patients on a particular ward are viewed negatively by staff and avoided by them. If these staff are forced to interact with these patients, for example to dispense medication, the interactions may be kept as brief as possible and are emotionally 'cool' or even hostile. Evidence of such staff hostility to patients who have assaulted them is provided by Cottle (1991). This atmosphere of 'social distance' between staff and patients on particular wards has also been linked to aggressive behaviour. Katz and Kirkland (1990) carried out a descriptive study of the organizational characteristics of violent wards.

> On wards identified as violent there was an atmosphere of fear and distrust and a sense of tension ... staff members rarely left the nursing station and conversations among patients were few and usually hostile ... The staff dealt with patients from inside a locked, glassed-in nursing station ... the psychiatrist rarely came on to the ward; one visit a day for a few minutes was not unusual. When the psychiatrists did come on the ward, they typically proceeded to the nursing station and ignored the patients ... Several avoided eye contact with

patients and ignored those patients who addressed them by name.

(Katz and Kirkland, 1990)

Again, it can be seen that the staff behaviour is more likely to be appraised as malicious or arbitrary by patients when it takes place in an atmosphere of social distance.

Furthermore, these two apparently opposing types of interaction, aversive stimulation and social distancing, may be most potent in causing aggression when they are combined. Maier *et al.* (1987) argue that the intrusive interactions such as frustration described above are more potentially dangerous when they take place within an overall ward atmosphere of social distance. Depp (1983) also proposes the importance of a combined effect of activity demands within a ward atmosphere characterized by staff who have withdrawn significant personal involvement and concern for patients.

Summary

Situational factors are likely to be important contributors to the occurrence of violent behaviour in psychiatric hospitals. Two opposing types of staff–patient interaction are seen as particularly relevant, especially when they occur together. These are aversive stimulation (angering the patient by physical or verbal intrusiveness or frustration) and social distancing (reducing the quantity and quality of interactions with patients).

STAFF INTERVENTIONS FOR POTENTIAL OR ACTUAL VIOLENCE

Potential or actual violence is a 'psychiatric emergency' that almost always calls for some sort of response from staff. For instance, only 1% aggressive incidents studied by Colenda and Hamer (1991) did not result in some sort of staff intervention. Interventions may range from 'counselling' and increased supervision of the patient to physical restraint, seclusion and medication (orally or intravenously, with or without the patient's consent). These interventions are often used in combination, starting with the least intrusive (e.g. talking to the patient) and introducing more intrusive and controlling measures as necessary (Pilowsky *et al.*, 1992). Most incidents of violence are dealt with by one or two nursing staff (Noble and Rodger, 1989) and only in more serious incidents are nurses from other wards or medical staff called in to provide assistance. It is noteworthy that police are rarely called to assist with the immediate management of violence in psychiatric hospitals but there is growing argument for use of legal sanctions in the long-term management of aggressive individuals where this is appropriate (Hoge and Gutheil, 1987).

While the interventions available to staff are well-known, there have been few attempts to evaluate which strategies are most effective, since controlled studies are difficult to conduct in this area. The use of physical restraint is known to be associated with staff injury (Carmel and Hunter, 1989). The administration of 'as required' (PRN) medication has received the most investigation. Pilowsky *et al.* (1992) examined 'rapid tranquillization' in response to violent behaviour and report that haloperidol and diazepam were the most commonly used drugs for sedation. Staff satisfaction was highest where this combination was used and patients who received it were less likely to require a second injection. McLaren *et al.* (1990) found that PRN medication was most commonly given in a secure unit to prevent or contain aggressive behaviour. Other interventions such as talking to or distracting the patient were used before and after the medication so that PRN 'formed the 'filling' of the sandwich of nursing interventions' (p. 733). There was a significant reduction in patient disturbance within 30 minutes and 70% of medicated patients had 'settled' within 1 hour.

CONCLUSIONS

This chapter was concerned initially with the 'epidemiology' of violence and then moved on to consider the types of patient who are more likely to engage in violent behaviour. This research will have some positive benefits for health care professionals since the accuracy of identifying which patients present the greatest risk is continually improving. However, it has been argued here that the next stage of research into violence in psychiatric hospitals should focus on situational factors such as frustration and intrusiveness, which are known to increase the likelihood of aggression by humans, regardless of mental disorder. These factors could then be combined with information on the types of individuals most at risk of becoming aggressive for a more complete explanation of violence in psychiatric hospitals. Future research could also examine the role of patient appraisals of staff behaviour as a factor in aggression.

REFERENCES

Adler, W., Kreeger, C. and Zeegler, P. (1983) Patient violence in a private psychiatric hospital, in *Assaults Within Psychiatric Facilities*, (eds J.R. Lion and W.H. Reid), Grune and Stratton, New York.

Aiken, G.J.M. (1984) Assaults on staff in a locked ward: prediction and consequences. *Medicine, Science and the Law*, **24**, 199–207.

Archer, J. (1989) From the laboratory to the community: studying the natural history of human aggression, in *Human Aggression: Naturalistic Approaches*, (eds J. Archer and K. Brown), Routledge, London.

Armond, A.D. (1982) Violence in the semi-secure ward of a psychiatric hospital. *Medicine, Science and the Law*, **22**, 203–209.

Blomhoff, S., Seim, S. and Friis, S. (1990) Can prediction of violence among psychiatric inpatients be improved? *Hospital and Community Psychiatry*, **41**, 771–75.

Carmel, H. and Hunter, M. (1989) Staff injuries from inpatient violence. *Hospital and Community Psychiatry*, **40**, 41–46.

COHSE (1976) *The Management of Violent and Potentially Violent Patients*. Confederation of Health Service Employees, Banstead.

Colenda, C.C. and Hamer, R.M. (1991) Antecedents and interventions for aggressive behaviour of patients in a geropsychiatric state hospital. *Hospital and Community Psychiatry*, **42**, 287–92.

Convey, J. (1986) A record of violence. *Nursing Times*, **82**(46), 36–38.

Convit, A., Jaeger, J., PinLin, S. *et al.* (1988) Predicting assaultiveness in psychiatric patients: a pilot study. *Hospital and Community Psychiatry*, **39**, 429–34.

Cooper, A.J. and Medonca, J.D. (1991) A prospective study of patient assaults on nurses in a provincial psychiatric hospital in Canada. *Acta Psychiatrica Scandinavica*, **84**, 163–66.

Cooper, S.J., Browne, F.W.A., McClean, K.J. *et al.* (1983) Aggressive behaviour in a psychiatric observation ward. *Acta Psychiatrica Scandinavica*, **68**, 386–93.

Cottle, M. (1991) *Expressed Emotion and Coping in Staff who have been Victims of Violence*. Paper presented at the Annual Conference of the British Psychological Society, Bournemouth, April 1991.

Cutting, J. (1981) Judgement of facial expression in schizophrenics. *British Journal of Psychiatry*, **139**, 1–6.

Davis, S. (1991) Violence by psychiatric inpatients: a review. *Hospital and Community Psychiatry*, **42**, 585–90.

Depp, F.C. (1983) Violent behavior patterns on psychiatric wards. *Aggressive Behavior*, **2**, 295–306.

DHSS (1976) *Management of Violent and Potentially Violent Hospital Patients*, HC(76)11, DHSS, London.

DHSS (1986) *Report of DHSS Conference on Violence to Staff*, DHSS, London.

DHSS (1988) *Violence to Staff. Report of the DHSS Advisory Committee on Violence to Staff*, HMSO, London.

Dooley, E. (1986) Aggressive incidents in a Secure Hospital. *Medicine, Science and Law*, **26**, 125–30.

Drinkwater, J. (1982) Violence in psychiatric hospitals, in *Developments in the Study of Criminal Behaviour. Vol. 2: Violence.* (ed. P. Feldman), John Wiley, Chichester.

Edwards, J.G., Jones, D., Reid, W.H. *et al.* (1988) Physical assaults in a psychiatric unit in a general hospital. *American Journal of Psychiatry*, **145**, 1568–1571.

Ekblom, B. (1970) *Acts of Violence by Patients in Mental Hospitals*, (translated by Helen Frey), Svenska Bokforlaget, Uppsala, Sweden.

Fottrell, E. (1980) A study of violent behaviour among patients in psychiatric hospitals. *British Journal of Psychiatry*, **136**, 216–21.

Geen, R.G. (1990) *Human Aggression*, Open University Press, Milton Keynes.

Haller, R.M. and Deluty, R.H. (1988) Assaults on staff by psychiatric inpatients. A critical review. *British Journal of Psychiatry*, **152**, 174–79.

Health Services Advisory Committee (1987) *Violence to Staff in the Health Services*, HMSO, London.

Hodgkinson, P.E., McIvor, L. and Phillips, M. (1985) Patient assaults on staff in a psychiatric hospital: a 2-year retrospective study. *Medicine, Science and the Law*, **25**, 288–94.

Hoge, S.K. and Gutheil, T.G. (1987) The prosecution of psychiatric patients for assaults on staff: a preliminary empirical study. *Hospital and Community Psychiatry*, **38**, 44–49.

Howells, K. (1982) Mental disorder and violent behaviour, in *Developments in the Study of Criminal Behaviour: Vol. 2: Violence*, (ed. P. Feldman), John Wiley, Chichester.

James, D.V., Fineberg, N.A., Shah, A.K. *et al.* (1990) An increase in violence on an acute psychiatric ward. A study of associated factors. *British Journal of Psychiatry*, **156**, 846–52.

Katz, P. and Kirkland, F.R. (1990) Violence and social structure on mental hospital wards. *Psychiatry*, **53**, 262–77.

Kronberg, M.E. (1983) Nursing intervention in the management of the assaultive patient, in *Assaults Within Psychiatric Facilities*, (eds J.R. Lion and W.H. Reid), Grune and Stratton, New York, pp. 225–40.

Lanza, M. (1983) The reactions of nursing staff to physical assault by a patient. *Hospital and Community Psychiatry*, **34**, 44–47.

Lanza, M.L. and Milner, J. (1989) The dollar cost of patient assault. *Hospital and Community Psychiatry*, **40**, 1227–29.

Larkin, E., Murtagh, S. and Jones, S. (1988) A preliminary study of violent incidents in a Special Hospital (Rampton). *British Journal of Psychiatry*, **153**, 226–31.

Lazarus, R. and Folkman, S. (1984) *Stress, Appraisal and Coping*, Springer, New York.

Lion, J.R. and Reid, W.H. (eds) (1983) *Violence Within Psychiatric Facilities*, Grune and Stratton, New York.

Lion, J.R., Snyder, W. and Merrill, G.L. (1981) Under-reporting of assaults on staff in a state hospital. *Hospital and Community Psychiatry*, **32**, 497–98.

Lowenstein, M., Binder, R.L. and McNiel, D.E. (1990) The relationship between admission symptoms and hospital assaults. *Hospital and Community Psychiatry*, **41**, 311–13.

Maier, G.J., Stava, L.J., Morrow, B.R. *et al.* (1987) A model for understanding and managing cycles of aggression among psychiatric inpatients. *Hospital and Community Psychiatry*, **38**, 520–24.

McLaren, S., Browne, F.W.A. and Taylor, P.J. (1990) A study of psychotropic medication given 'as required' in a Regional Secure Unit. *British Journal of Psychiatry*, **156**, 732–35.

Noble, P. and Rodger, S. (1989) Violence by psychiatric inpatients. *British Journal of Psychiatry*, **155**, 384–90.

Owens, R.G. and Bagshaw, M. (1985) First steps in the functional analysis of aggression, in *Current Issues in Clinical Psychology*, (ed. E. Karaf), Plenum Press, London, pp. 285–307.

Pearson, M., Wilmot, E. and Padi, M. (1986) A study of violent behaviour among inpatients in a psychiatric hospital. *British Journal of Psychiatry*, **149**, 232–35.

Pilowsky, L.S., Ring, H., Shine, P.J. *et al.* (1992) Rapid tranquillization: A survey of emergency prescribing in a general psychiatric hospital. *British Journal of Psychiatry*, **160**, 831–35.

Poyner, B. and Warne, C. (1986) *Violence to Staff. A Basis for Assessment and Prevention*, HMSO, London.

Roscoe, J. (1987) *Survey on the Incidence and Nature of Violence Occurring in the Joint Hospitals. Report to the Bethlem Royal and Maudsley Hospitals Special Health Authority Working Party on Violence.*

Ryan, J.A. and Poster, E.C. (1989) The assaulted nurse: short-term and long-term responses. *Archives of Psychiatric Nursing*, **3**, 323–31.

Saunders, L. (1991) *Safe and Secure in Surrey. Research into Violence to Social Services Staff.* Paper presented at the Annual Conference of the British Psychological Society, Bournemouth, April 1991.

Sheridan, M., Henrion, R., Robinson, L. *et al.* (1990) Precipitants of violence in a psychiatric inpatient setting. *Hospital and Community Psychiatry*, **41**, 776–80.

Tardiff, K. and Sweillam, A. (1982) Assaultive behaviour among chronic inpatients. *American Journal of Psychiatry*, **139**, 212–15.

Walker, E., McGuire, M. and Bettes, B. (1984) Recognition and identification of facial stimuli by schizophrenics and patients with affective disorders. *British Journal of Clinical Psychiatry*, **23**, 37–44.

Walmsley, R. (1986) *Personal Violence*. Home Office Research and Planning Unit Report. Home Office Research Study No. 89, HMSO, London.

Whittington, R. and Wykes, T. (1992) Staff strain and social support in a psychiatric hospital following assault by a patient. *Journal of Advanced Nursing*, **17**, 480–86.

CHAPTER 3

Violence to social workers

Stanley Bute

INTRODUCTION

Social workers have never had the positive public image that some other professions enjoy. For example, when 25-year-old Police Constable Yvonne Fletcher was murdered while carrying out police duty in April 1984, the media quite rightly brought the matter to the immediate attention of the public. Few people could have missed the newspaper headlines or television's graphic account of the incident. However, when Norma Morris became the second social worker to be murdered within a matter of a few months, one of her former colleagues expressed views that were strongly held by many others in the profession:

> Had the social worker, Norma Morris, been a police woman I suspect that the national papers would have told the nation of this tragedy. Had Ms. Morris been accused of neglecting a client, it might well have been broadcast nationally.
>
> *(Barnett, 1985)*

Haringey's Director of Social Services also commented that:

> Social Services staff are used by society as agents of social care and control. They are charged not only to protect individuals ... from society, but also to protect society and themselves from those same individuals. Unlike the police, they wear no uniforms and carry no weapons: but they do have a much more complicated job. They are required, on occasions, for example, forcibly to remove children from parents, to admit to psychiatric hospitals, and to supervise young people whose behaviour has brought them before the courts ... They do this work willingly. But the extent to which their work is subject to unbalanced criticism is both unreasonable and unworthy. It is thoroughly demoralizing. Social Services staff do not expect to be regarded as saints or the

epitome of efficiency. They know they are neither. But they sometimes risk and give their lives in helping people whom society has rejected. They have a right to expect a recognition of the value of what they do.

(Townsend, 1985)

At the DHSS conference on violence to staff convened by Norman Fowler on 2 December 1986, David Jones announced that, with the Secretary of State and 800 others, he had the previous day attended a memorial service in Birmingham for the life of Frances Bettridge.

It was unacceptable that an event of such importance had not been recognized by the television news programmes.

(Jones, 1986)

One wonders whether and to what extent the sympathies of the media and public lie with the sentiments expressed by Geoffrey Dickens. In a debate in the House of Commons on the subject of violence towards social workers, he said:

Is it not true that there are recruited into the social services many odd bods who are long-haired, unshaven, and who wear political badges on their lapels, who provoke attacks upon themselves by their very attitude?

(Hansard, 1986)

FREQUENCY OF VIOLENCE IN SOCIAL WORK

Until the late 1970s, violence does not appear to have been a significant problem for members of the social work profession. Relieving officers, duly authorized officers, and then mental welfare officers would undoubtedly have experienced occasional violence or the threat of such when carrying out their responsibilities under the relevant mental health legislation of their day. However, these incidents seem to have gone unreported.

It took several years for members of the social work profession to realize that violence to staff was increasing at a rate that could not be ignored and to such an extent that it had to be dealt with on a professional basis. Inevitably, as members of the profession were killed during the course of their work, staff expressed an increasing concern and demand for action from employers.

Peter Gray, a social worker, was stabbed to death by a client when visiting the man in the Shirley area of Southampton on 4 July 1978.

Isabel Schwarz died in her office on 6 July 1984 at Bexley Psychiatric Hospital: she was killed by a former client.

Norma Morris died in April 1985 while visiting a youth who had tried to commit suicide in Haringey, London.

Frances Bettridge was murdered on 5 September 1986 while visiting the home of a client in Birmingham.

Richard Kirkman, a residential social worker, was stabbed to death at a hostel for single homeless people in May 1987 in Stockport.

Alan Whittall was an Intermediate Treatment worker in Manchester before he was murdered in 1987.

If these have been the worst cases of violence during recent years, they are the 'worst' only because the victims have all died. Many other social workers have been attacked and have the effects of horrific assaults. Many incidents have been unreported and are, therefore, unknown; several others have been reported in the professional press.

Murray Bruggen, a probation officer, received brain damage following an attack that took place in his office in November 1974.

Arthur Caiger, also a probation officer, became blind on 1 December 1978 following an assault by a man who threw hydrochloric acid into his face.

Pat Watling, a female probation officer, was stabbed by a drug-abusing client during a home visit in 1978.

Peter Durrant was severely injured in 1985 in a road traffic accident while trying to escort a patient to psychiatric hospital. The accident happened when the patient attempted to grab the steering wheel of the car, which was being driven by a police officer.

Peter Gray died in Southampton in 1978. Shortly before Gray's death, also in Southampton, S.F. Bute had personally experienced being unlawfully imprisoned and threatened by a client whose two children had been taken into care. These two events motivated Bute to make representation to members of the social work profession (Bute, 1979a). The representation called for guidelines that would help social workers prevent violent incidents and assist in managing situations when things went wrong. On professional training courses it appeared that many were being taught to 'casework' violence rather than retreat from it. That cry for help produced no overt response and so, using a DHSS circular (Department of Health and Social Security, 1976) as a guide, Bute produced what was probably the first booklet of its kind with a stated objective of helping social workers in the prevention and management of violence (Bute, 1980). No one could have predicted the subsequent phenomenal demand for copies from social services and health organizations throughout the country and overseas. From then onwards, the need for guidelines was never in question.

Hampshire cannot be described as a county that experiences an above average amount of violence by clients. However, recent monitoring of incidents in Hampshire County Council (i.e. not only social services) showed that one member of staff is physically abused or threatened every 2 hours. Employees request counselling in approximately 10% of serious incidents. Examples include attacks by gangs of youths (education), assault and injury by clients with mental health problems (social services), threats to an employee's children (social services), and repeated arson attacks (libraries) (Hampshire Social Services, 1991a). This level of violence is likely to be experienced in other parts of the country but there is still no consistent approach to the problem.

Research studies

During the past few years a few studies have been published in an attempt to gain a better understanding of violence by clients towards staff. One of the problems experienced in the investigation of what precipitates violent incidents and how they can be prevented is that the definitions and methods of collating statistical information show considerable variation between departments. This makes it very difficult, if not impossible, for objective analysis of data. In this chapter, an abbreviated summary will be presented in chronological order. The headings will indicate the researcher's definition of violence, the method used, and the study's main findings. Even if statistical comparisons cannot be made, a consideration of the main issues can be addressed by identifying shared concerns.

Wessex (1979) study

A postal survey carried out in Wessex (Brown *et al.*, 1986) revealed that most attacks upon fieldworkers occurred when they were undertaking statutory duties. Cited examples were those of removing a child into care or escorting a psychiatric patient to hospital in circumstances when the patient had no desire to be admitted. Even admission of elderly, confused people to residential care under the provisions of the National Assistance Act had its occasional problems. Many authorities now make use of legislation that enables guardianship to be used in place of section 47 of the National Assistance Act. This obviates the necessity to apply to a court for the removal of the elderly person. However, it does not remove the potential for violence, even though this is more likely to be limited to aggression rather than dangerousness.

Definition

In this study, violence was defined as actual physical assault resulting in some injury or pain and violence to property that involved actual damage.

Method

A questionnaire was sent to 560 staff working in personal social services in Wessex (contacted through professional organizations). Of those contacted, 338 replied.

Main findings

The main findings of the study were that the level of violence was higher than expected. Several staff experienced at least one violent incident in the previous 3 years of the current post (Table 3.1). The precipitating factors to violence were as follows:

- deprivation of personal liberty;
- social control (i.e. children into care/compulsory admission of mentally disordered persons);
- withholding information or services;
- giving advice or disciplining a client in a residential home or day centre; and
- intervening to protect a third party.

Table 3.1 Staff in various settings with experience of at least one violent incident in previous 3 years of current post

	Number assaulted	Number in sample	Percentage assaulted
Day centre	22	44	50
Residential	32	71	45
Field	39	177	22
Other	5	21	24
Administrative	0	20	0
Total	98	333	29

Although the Wessex research project had some design limitations, the unavoidable and significant conclusion was that violence was perceived as a problem by social workers in Wessex and that they wanted something done about it. Many wanted to be properly trained to prevent violence, others asked for the problem to be acknowledged by their managers. Most of the respondents (89% of the 44 day centre workers, 90% of the 71 residential staff, and 85% of the 177 fieldworkers) felt there should be printed guidelines for the management of violence.

Rowett 1983/1984 study

As a research study of violence in the context of local authority social work, Rowett's work (Rowett, 1986) was an important contribution to the on-going debate.

In this study, violence was defined as physical (including sexual) violence resulting in actual physical harm to the social worker (SWR). Threats, abuse, or any other form of psychological violence were excluded. The method was as follows:

1. A questionnaire was sent to all 132 social services departments (SSDs) – the response was 31%.
2. A scanning questionnaire was then sent to all SWRs (728) in one shire county SSD – the response was 62%.
3. Structured interviews ($n = 120$) of a sample from the shire county results (60 SWRs who were assaulted matched with 60 nonassaulted colleagues). 343 (76%) respondents to the scanning survey agreed to be interviewed to discuss in more detail their views and experiences of violent clients. 30 assaulted field social workers (FSWs) and 30 assaulted residential social workers (RSWs) were chosen and matched with nonassaulted colleagues from the respective sectors.

Main findings
These were as follows:

1. Stage 1 (National survey)
   (a) The absolute number of recorded incidents increased steadily during the 5 year period 1978–1982 (Table 3.2). This could have reflected a genuine increase in assaults, or greater awareness and recording of incidents.
   (b) A little more than two-thirds of the local authority SSDs in England, Wales, Scotland and Northern Ireland did not complete the questionnaire.
   (c) RSWs were appreciably more likely to be assaulted than FSWs.
   (d) Senior managers in the survey considered that the rate of recorded violence was tolerable and acceptable.
   (e) Several authorities pointed out that there was an acknowledged shortfall between actual and reported incidents. Few SSDs collated the information they collected.
2. Stage 2 (Scanning survey)
   (a) RSWs were more likely to be assaulted than FSWs.
   (b) There was a disparity between the incidence rate projected from the national survey and the recorded incidence rate. If the national incidence rate for shire counties had been adopted,

five SWRs should have been assaulted during the survey period for a sample of 450. In fact, 112 SWRs (25%) reported at least one assault, while 40% of all the SWRs who had been assaulted stated that they had been assaulted on more than one occasion.

(c) Most SWRs are women: most assaulted SWRs are men.

(d) Of officer grade RSWs, 51% had been assaulted on more than one occasion.

3. Stage 3 (Structured interviews)

(a) Of the sample, 74 (62%) were aged 40 years or younger.

(b) The 60 SWRs were physically assaulted a total of 588 times in a 6-year period (1978–1983), an average of 1.6 assaults per SWR per year.

(c) Most of these incidents were minor and would have involved slaps, punches, and scratches that were sufficient to inflict physical harm but probably not involving medical, other than first aid, treatment.

(d) The number of assaults on individual SWRs differed widely. Three female RSWs were, between them, assaulted 256 times (120, 90, 46 assaults, respectively) and three male RSWs were assaulted a total of 121 times (48, 42, 31 assaults, respectively). If these six are excluded, the remaining 54 SWRs were assaulted 3.9 times on average; this would result in an average of 0.7 assaults per SWR per year.

Table 3.2 Assaulted social workers 1978–1982[a]

| | 1978 | | 1979 | | 1980 | | 1981 | | 1982 | | Total |
	F	R	F	R	F	R	F	R	F	R	12
SWRs physically injured requiring at least 4 weeks sick leave	0	1	0	0	1	3	0	1	2	6	14
SWRs requesting compensatory leave after a violent assault	0	1	0	5	0	3	1	2	1	6	19
SWRs seeking financial compensation under CICB scheme	0	0	0	0	1	3	0	4	1	3	12
SWRs needing medical treatment after a physical assault	8	35	17	44	20	69	26	92	21	111	443

[a] Abbreviations: SWR = social worker; F = field social worker; R = residential social worker; CICB = Criminal Injuries Compensation Board.

Rowett observed that:

> From the interviews with the 60 assaulted SWRs it was apparent that the incidence rate for assault indicated by the scanning survey and the national survey represented only a small proportion of the actual number of assaults during the survey period.
>
> *(Rowett, 1986)*

The problem of under-reporting/under-recording is an important issue and one to which more attention must be given.

There were 588 incidents in the reported total. Rowett acknowledges a skewed distribution created by the presence of the six heavily assaulted SWRs, but he considered that ' . . . even if the assaults on those six are excluded, the remaining total is sufficiently high to give cause for concern'. Rowett conjectured that it may be the case that most SWRs in SSDs in any one year are harmed by clients at least once, sufficient to cause bruising or more serious physical damage.

Most assaults were on RSWs. More RSWs were assaulted frequently. Female RSWs are most frequently assaulted. The average age of the assaultive client was 31.9 years, with a range of 10–85 years. Of the assaultive clients 43% were under the age of 18 years. The most common assailants of RSWs are shown in Table 3.3.

Table 3.3 Age of assaultive client by group

Age of client (years)	18	19–30	31–40	41–50	51–60	+60	Total
Assaulted FSWR	8	6	8	5	2	1	30
Assaulted RSWR	18	2	2	1	1	6	30
Total	26	8	10	6	3	7	60
Percentage	43	13	17	10	5	12	100

More than one in four of the assaultive clients had a conviction for violence. In both field and residential contexts, the aggressive clients were usually smaller or the same size as their SWRs. Rowett commented that it is difficult to evaluate the data on the explanations for violence with any confidence. Nine SWRs could not explain the violent incident and many 'reasons' bore little or no relationship to the descriptions of what actually happened before and during the actual incidents.

Approximately one-fifth of the managers were never informed of the assault. This might be related to the fact that of the nonassaulted SWRs most considered 'incompetence' as a characteristic of assaulted colleagues. Assaulted social workers presumably do not want to be accused of not being good at their job so keep quiet. Of the managers who were informed, 33% provided a response that the social worker did not find satisfactory. Only a little over half of the incidents resulted in a satisfactory managerial response (Table 3.4). The major source of support came from colleagues.

Table 3.4 Responses from managers by group[a]

Group	Did not inform	Told manager: satisfactory response	Told manager: unsatisfactory response	Total
AFSW	6	17	7	30
ARSW	5	16	9	30
Total	11	33	16	60
Percentage	18	55	27	100

[a]Abbreviations: AFSW = assaulted field social worker; ARSW = assaulted residential social worker.

Most of the 60 assaulted social workers were unaware that they could have claimed compensation from their employer or the Criminal Injuries Compensation Board scheme.

Rowett concluded that, with adequate training, and the development of management information-feedback systems, the incidence rate could be reduced and the consequence of assault for SWRs much improved.

Strathclyde (1987)

In Scotland, a well researched document was published as a result of the deliberations of a joint working party consisting of trade union members and departmental staff (Strathclyde Regional Council, 1987). In the autumn of 1985, there had been an incident at the Wallacewell children's home in Glasgow in which a member of staff was attacked by a 14-year-old boy. This led to a bitter dispute between staff and management that eventually affected nearly half the region's children's homes. One of the positive results of the dispute was an agreement to form the working party.

The comprehensive report was produced in only 6 months and, in addition to a detailed analysis of a written response from staff throughout the authority, consultations took place with external departments and organizations that contributed valuable information and expertise.

Definition of violence
Purposeful or reactive behaviour intended to produce damaging or hurtful effects, physically or emotionally, on other persons.

Method
Monitoring exercise to identify the extent and nature of violence in work places in Strathclyde. Incidents in 20 residential units, 16 fieldwork units and 17 day care units were monitored and reported on a standard form from 1st October to 30th November 1985.

Main findings
A breakdown of the results of the monitoring exercise is given in Table 3.5.

Table 3.5 Summary of incidents in Strathclyde establishments[a]

Type of establishment	Number of incidents	Units reporting: monitored	Type of assault: Physical violence	Verbal abuse	Physical posturing
Area team	7	6:16	1	4	2
Day care	7	4:17	6	1	0
Children's home	30	7: 8	17	?	?
Assessment centre	21	2: 2	15	?	?
Residence for elderly people	11	4: 6	7	4	0
Residence for handicapped people	2	2: 4	0	2	0

[a]N.B. Not all reported incidents were directed at staff: 3 incidents in the area teams were directed at clerical staff; in the residential units for people with a handicap, the violence was client to client.

For the assessment centres there was a large difference in reporting. This is likely to be due partly to a different perception of, and level of concern about, violence in the two institutions and should not be seen to indicate that the residents in one were more violent than those in the other.

The report concludes with a general comment that, from the responses to the exercise, most incidents did not fit with the report's definition in that violence could not have been described as intentional.

Surrey 1987 study (Saunders, 1987)

In the same year, Surrey Social Services undertook and published a survey of all front-line staff and their managers or supervisors (Surrey County Council, 1987).

Definition of violence
Any situation where a client exhibits behaviour that is deemed disruptive, dangerous to staff, to other clients or to property. Specific definitions were as follows:

1. *Physical assault*: assault, with or without a weapon, resulting in actual physical harm to the member of staff at the level of bruising/cuts/hair-pulling, or more serious injury.
2. *Physical abuse*: attempted assault with or without a weapon that did not result in actual physical harm to the member of staff.
3. *Sexual assault*: resulting in actual physical harm to the member of staff at the level of bruising/cuts/lacerations or more serious injury.
4. *Sexual abuse*: sexual harrassment or other forms of inappropriate sexual behaviour that did not result in actual physical harm to the member of staff.
5. *Threats*: verbal or written, to the person or to property, or both.
6. *Property damage or thefts*: of the property of the member of staff, including leased cars as personal property.
7. *Other*: any form of physical (including sexual) assault, or psychological abuse, or threats, not contained in the above, which the member of staff considers to have been sufficiently serious to warrant concern.

Method

A survey was made of all front-line staff and their managers or supervisors in three stages:

1. Scanning questionnaire was sent to 4055 staff. Of these 1570 (39%) responded: 528 had experienced violence. Of these, 263 indicated their willingness to answer more detailed questions.
2. Second questionnaire to the 263 willing respondents. Different questionnaires were sent to staff who had experienced different types of violence (see definitions) over the 5 years to 1 December 1986. In all, 601 forms were sent out. The response rate varied according to the type of violence.
3. A personal interview was conducted with 20 staff. (Interviewees were selected to ensure that every type of violence and a variety of workbases were represented.)

Main findings

Of the 528 who had experienced violence in some form during the 5-year period covered by the study, 301 staff members had experienced more than one type of violence (Figure 3.1). One person reported experiencing six types of violence.

Most assaults on fieldworkers occurred in the client's home or, interestingly, when interviewing patients in hospital. Rowett's concern about under-reporting was matched by the Surrey study in that a significant number of incidents were unreported or reported only to colleagues (presumbly peers). Line managers would, therefore,

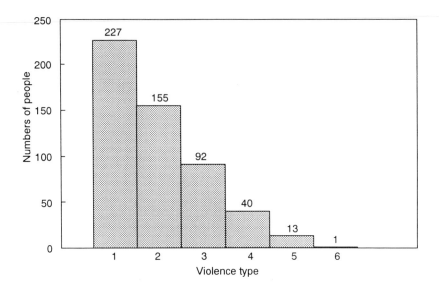

Figure 3.1 Number of people experiencing combinations of violent types.

have been unaware of the unreported incidents. Reported incidents were often not recorded on the appropriate accident form and, therefore, were not lodged centrally. Of those reported to line managers, approximately 35% of the respondents considered that they had not received an adequate response from that person. Given this finding, together with the clear reluctance to inform management at any level, more thought needs to be given to the ways in which managers should respond when violence occurs.

The most common form of violence was a threat (327 people), while 261 experienced physical abuse, 208 physical assault, 108 damage to or theft of property, 59 sexual abuse, and four sexual assault (two men and two women). There were 77 'other' cases (Figure 3.2).

Commenting on the results of the scanning survey, the report states that:

The responses received suggest that violence is more prevalent than originally thought – occurring within all work bases, in all types of job, to all age groups, and both sexes – and with over a third of the respondents having experienced it in some form ... Certain work contexts appear to be more vulnerable to incidents of violence than others, most notably community homes, homes for elderly people, hostels and day centres for

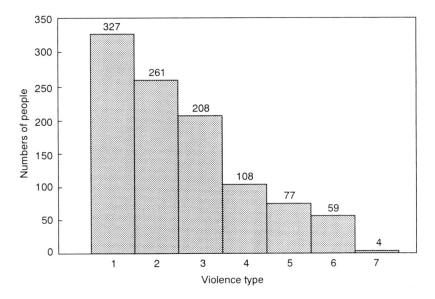

Figure 3.2 Number of people experiencing each type of violence: 1=threat; 2=physical abuse; 3=physical assault; 4=property damage/theft; 5=other; 6=sexual abuse; 7=sexual assault.

handicapped people ... Field social work staff are less likely to experience violence ... This does fit with previous research that has found that although the incidence is higher in residential social work, the consequences of violence in field social work have generally been more serious.

The number of respondents experiencing each type of violence at least once is shown in Figure 3.2.

In this study, 528 had reported an experience of violence: only 263 of these respondents (49%) indicated a willingness to provide more information. 601 forms were sent out and only 240 were returned (Table 3.6).

Many serious threats were directed at staff. The more serious the threat, the less likely was the line manager to be informed. The data did not identify what proportion of the threats, if any, resulted in the threatened action taking place.

Stage 3 of the study (20 interviews) revealed that verbal abuse from clients appeared to be an accepted part of the social work task. Workers were most vulnerable when visiting clients with no prior information, taking a child into care and being involved in formal psychiatric admissions to hospital. These findings reflect those of the much earlier Wessex study. Even when records of a client's threatening behaviour existed, workers did not always take precautions. Line managers

Table 3.6 Type of violence experienced

Type of violence	Question-naires sent	Question-naires returned	Return rate (%)	Line manager informed (%)	Satisfactory response from line manager
Physical assault	132	57	43.2	70.2	64.0
Physical abuse	149	63	38.2	73.1	70.0
Sexual assault	5	0	–	–	–
Sexual abuse	32	12	37.5	75.0	66.6
Threat	181	82	45.3	53.9	64.7
Property damage/theft	63	21	33.3	66.6	60.0
Other	39	5	12.8	–	–
Total	601	240	39.9		

were criticized for not taking incidents seriously, a lack of sensitivity in dealing with workers after incidents, not changing practice as a result of incidents and avoiding important issues arising from incidents.

University of Sussex study (Kedward, 1990)

Definition of violence

Not indicated. The author of the study makes the point that the questionnaire was designed to yield the maximum information with the least expenditure of time and resources on the part of the respondents. The purpose of the study was to obtain a general picture of practice with regard to violence.

Method

In March 1989, questionnaires were sent to all directors of social services (132) and chief probation officers (56) in the UK with an accompanying letter asking for their help. From the directors, 71 replies were received, of which 60 (45.5%) were usable. Of the chief probation officers 33 replied; only 19 (33.9%) were usable.

Main findings

The main findings from the responses received from the social services were:

1. There is a need to standardize data collection.
2. Detailed surveys tend to reveal much higher levels of violence than expected.
3. Insufficient information is available in relation to threats of violence.
4. Several departments appear to have no coherent policy in relation to violence.

Kedward's questionnaire was intentionally straightforward and easy to respond to in order to elicit a good response. Therefore a question asking for information about recording incidents was of a general nature and did not attempt to obtain a substantial breakdown of figures that would indicate trends of violence towards social workers. However, the author was able to conclude that:

What is immediately clear from even these basic figures and the accompanying letters is that the problem of violence for social workers is a real one, is not confined to certain areas with particular problems, is more serious than had previously been realized and is increasing, though at what rate is difficult to determine.

(Kedward, 1990)

As already noted, Rowett had expressed similar concern (Rowett, 1986). This important issue will also be discussed when the responsibilities of employers are considered.

These concerns are justifiable. Very few social services departments appear to record incidents of staff being **threatened** by violence. Kedward draws attention to the death of Isabel Schwarz and the Department of Health and Social Security's (DHSS) *Report of the Committee of Inquiry into the Care and Aftercare of Miss Sharon Campbell* (DHSS, 1988). On 22 August 1985, Miss Campbell became the subject of a Court Order under Section 51 of the Mental Health Act 1983, having been found not mentally fit to stand trial for the murder of Isabel Schwarz. Direct threats and threatening telephone calls had been made to Ms Schwarz during the 6-month period of October 1983 to March 1984. Their significance appears to have been underestimated with devastating results. The DHSS report recommended that social workers should be trained and instructed to report incidents of violence **and threats of violence** (emphasis added) and that employing authorities should issue written guidelines on the method of reporting them. As long ago as December 1979, attention had been drawn (Bute, 1979b) to the **threat** of violence by clients, which, as the Wessex Study showed (Brown *et al.*, 1986), can be as great a problem as actual assault because, generally, it happens more frequently and yet can be just as disabling.

Community care issues

Dooley (1988) drew attention to the increasing problem of managing potentially violent patients in the community as a result of the trend towards closing large psychiatric hospitals in favour of small establishments and family type units. Dooley's words were prophetic for many authorities that have found it difficult to cope with extreme behaviour, which, previously, had been just about manageable with the help of hospital procedures and therapy. In Hampshire (Hampshire Social Services, 1990), for example, incidents of violence increased significantly in one geographical area of the county during the 3-month period July to September 1990. It was noted that the area had absorbed many discharged patients from a local hospital for people with learning difficulties. However, it must also be said that Hampshire's statistics are not refined and could have been skewed by several factors. For example, it would appear that staff tend to be more aware of incident report forms (and are apparently more willing to complete them) immediately after completing a training course on violence. Nevertheless, the management of potentially violent patients in the community is a cause for concern for community social workers and care staff who are often working in isolation and one-to-one situations.

The community care issue cannot be ignored. It seems highly likely that it will become more pronounced during the next few years. Hudson has commented that:

> ... deinstitutionalization looks set to accelerate in the 1990's. Over the next 5 years, 24 hospitals for people with learning disabilities are planned to close with a loss of 2707 beds, and 36 psychiatric hospitals with 12 525 beds.
>
> (*Hudson, 1990*)

We must be careful to ensure that incidents of violence do not accelerate at the same rate.

RESPONSE OF EMPLOYERS

In some respects, it was brave of the Surrey department to publish its survey findings, which highlight criticisms of line managers. Managers were accused of not taking incidents seriously, lacking in sensitivity when relating to workers after incidents of violence, not changing practice as a result of incidents, and avoiding important issues arising from incidents. One residential social worker is even reported as having been told by a senior manager that assault was a professional hazard.

Although the Surrey report findings are based on a relatively small response rate (and is confined to a single county perspective), it makes some useful observations. For example, there is an overwhelming need for middle and senior managers to be seen as supportive. A huge bridge has to be crossed before some managers are **perceived** as supportive. Managers throughout the country must consider carefully how they relate to their staff. In many cases, attitudes will need to change. Seated behind the security of an office desk, it can be very easy for a manager to dismiss violence as an occupational hazard.

There are also practical undertakings that managers at all levels have to consider. Kedward (1990) was encouraged by the progress made by many authorities to respond appropriately in either emotional or practical ways. Peers were perceived as having an invaluable role in supporting colleagues who had suffered. In addition, many authorities had developed impressive ways in which to respond to the problem of violence. Some of these methods were selected by Kedward as being of interest to authorities who are not so far advanced in the provision of support arrangements:

> They include a London borough setting up a reciprocal scheme (to provide a sensitive personal response to victims) with other neighbouring boroughs; a shire county setting up a county-wide panel of professions; [and] a London borough using the county psychological service. Others mentioned funding a member of staff as specialist Counsellor or setting up a link with Relate.
>
> *(Kedward, 1990)*

These examples illustrate that much work has already been done. Some of the important practical issues, which, collectively, represent a minimum package with which all employers should start to formulate policies and a code of practice, will now be considered briefly. They include:

- reporting, recording and monitoring procedures;
- guidelines on the prevention and management of violence;
- work environments;
- training (including physical restraint);
- counselling; and
- compensation and prosecution.

Thorough consideration of these issues will not always prevent violence but if they are comprehensively addressed, workers at the sharp end are likely to feel safer. They will certainly feel more supported.

Reporting, recording and monitoring

Prior to 1983 very few social services departments had set up systems to record incidents of violence towards staff. Social workers were not actively encouraged to report assaults or the threat of such except in the general context of undertaking the formality of a brief reference in the 'accident book'. Rowett comments that 'under-recording would also seem to be substantially influenced by the attitudes of the assaulted social workers themselves and of their line managers' (Rowett, 1986).

One reason why Norris undertook the Nova study (Norris, 1990) was because of concern about under-reporting. His research sample was very small (38 respondents) but 32 (84%) agreed that social workers were reluctant to report client attacks to management. In that study most people suggested that the reluctance to report was because social workers felt they were to blame for the violence, and did not want to be seen by others as unskilled or inadequate.

A report published by the Local Government Management Board (Stockdale and Phillips, 1991) has also concluded that a significant proportion of violent incidents are not formally recorded. The report makes its statement following a study of procedures in two local authorities, Leicester City Council and Dorset County Council. A subsequent health and safety information bulletin commented that:

> ... a low level of reported incidents (of violence towards staff) may reflect a lack of awareness of the appropriate reporting procedures, rather than a low level of occurrence. The report estimates that, in the two Local Authorities studied, one in three incidents of violence or physical attack and two out of three incidents of aggressive or threatening behaviour are not formally recorded.
>
> (*Health and Safety Executive, 1991*)

Despite the negative connotations of the findings in these two geographical areas, it is worth noting that the social service departments in the two local authorities (Dorset Social Services and Leicestershire County Social Services) both have an outstanding record of progress made in terms of the production of guidelines and communication of the respective issues to staff members. In Dorset, an interim document was produced in 1986 pending the publication of a printed booklet the following year. In Leicestershire, a very comprehensive booklet was published in 1987. Strenuous attempts have since been made to address the problem through training initiatives and a range of working practices. The design of accommodation is accepted as a factor in the prevention of violence and progress has been made with necessary adaptations to premises. Design briefs for new premises are taking violence into consideration. If there is under-reporting by social workers in Leicestershire and Dorset, where much attention has been focused on the prevention and management of violence, one should be more than a little concerned about what is happening in social services departments that have failed to address the issue during recent years.

When the Health and Safety Executive (HSE) published a paper on violence to staff (Poyner and Warne, 1986), the authors included an extremely useful suggestion for the contents of an incident report form. Virtually the same form was produced in the following year by the Health and Safety Commission's Health Service Advisory Committee (Health Services Advisory Committee, 1987). Also in 1987, the Association of Directors of Social Services issued its invaluable '*Guidelines*' booklet, which, again, included a copy of the HSE Incident Report Form (Association of Directors of Social Services, 1987). This is the nearest one has come to a situation where health and social services organizations have had easy opportunity to use the same definitions, the same criteria, the same documentation, the same guidelines and procedures for recording and monitoring incidents that arise in our workplaces from time to time. Policy and practice have pushed us into ensuring that general accident reports are completed, so that staff know what is required of them when reporting and recording industrial injuries. It is surely not impossible that social service departments agree to the same definitions, so that the same questions can be asked and the same documentation used for recording and monitoring the incidence of violence. Only in this way will one be able to make meaningful progress towards being able to compare and learn from the resulting statistical evidence.

Guidelines

In the late 1970s it was very clear that social workers wanted their employers to provide support by producing guidelines that would help staff to prevent violence and enable them to respond professionally when an assault took place. Many authorities have now published their own guidelines. Some have, quite rightly, used material from other authorities. Others have taken the lead from comprehensive reports by organizations such as the ADSS (Association of Directors of Social Services, 1987), BASW (British Association of Social Workers, 1988) and the Health and Safety Commission (Health Services Advisory Committee, 1987). It is not appropriate to enter into an in-depth discussion about the necessary contents of guidelines. Some work has been performed on this subject (Johnson, 1987). The principles upon which to base a publication would certainly include a need for the document to be clear, concise, easily understood and comprehensive. Guidelines should be practical and feasible with a marked absence of bureaucratic language and a consistent underlining of the fact that management's intention is to be supportive – especially when things go wrong. Guidelines are best drawn up by a group of staff from all levels of the department. This becomes more difficult but not impossible in situations where codes of practice are collated by interdepartmental working groups (as in Hampshire County Council). However, even in these circumstances, an attempt should be made to involve practitioners. A collection of managers or advisers are likely to see things quite differently from staff who have responsibility for day-to-day contact with the department's customers. Trades union representation will also help to provide this important balance.

Work environment

Many social services departments have tried to give consideration to the environment in which social workers are employed and in which customers are received. Receptionists are in the front-line and among the first to receive an angry person's verbal onslaught. Directors should, therefore, carefully consider the need for a welcoming reception area. This applies to the decor and security arrangements rather than the calibre of reception staff. Many departments have provided good alarm systems for use in emergencies. Several have also ensured that all staff members are fully aware of the procedures to be followed in the event of the alarm being triggered. Further consideration will be given to this important issue in Chapter 12.

Training

General training

The report of the Association of Directors of Social Services recommended that training to deal with situations of violence should be examined in greater detail by the Central Council for Education and Training in Social Work and should be included in training course core curricula. The report went on to suggest that local authorities ought to focus attention on the subject in their own in-service/in-house training programmes (Association of Directors of Social Services, 1987). Some progress has been made by local authorities, universities and polytechnics, but it is disappointing that many social work students still receive very little, if any, training to prepare them for violent threats and encounters. Following a questionnaire to all Scottish courses, it was established (in February 1990) that only two CQSW and two CSS courses in Scotland dealt with the topic (Phillips and Leadbetter, 1990). Stirling University responded to the need by introducing a course that was to address comprehensively causes, prevention, and pre-/post-incident management of violence.

Physical restraint

While this is a subject to be considered more fully in Chapter 10, reference is made at this point because physical restraint has never been an easy option for social workers. However, there is little doubt that, on occasion and as a last resort, the technique has to be used, either for the safety of the social worker or to protect other people who are at risk of assault. It seems likely that staff who work in residential and day-care services will be called upon to use physical restraint techniques more frequently than their fieldwork colleagues. Nevertheless, most of the victims of the fatal incidents that have occurred in recent years have been fieldworkers so all members of the profession have to consider carefully their position. To avoid doing so could be courting disaster.

Experience shows that it takes time for social workers and their managers to come to terms with the need for staff to be trained in the proper use of restraint. There appear to be all sorts of inhibitions that may well stem from basic professional training. Some course organizers have included specific training on how to prevent and manage violence but, generally, this appears to stop short of the need for self-defence. 'What do I do when something goes wrong?' is a question that, for a long time, has not received a convincing reply. To retreat, to get out and get away, is certainly a good idea if that is, in any way, a possibility. There will nevertheless be occasions when one has to stand one's ground.

In Hampshire, general training programmes aim to help staff prevent and manage violence. After much thought and discussion, in April 1987, Hampshire's departmental working group recommended the Director's management team to allow and provide training for **passive** self-defence such as holding or restraining a violent person. In June 1991, as a supplement to the Hampshire Code of Practice, a practice guidance booklet was published for all social service staff (Hampshire Social Services, 1991b). The Hampshire document also helps to clarify what the authors perceive to be the criteria for restraint:

> A member of staff may restrain a client when that person has directed towards themselves or another: (i) aggressive physical contact that may or may not result in pain or injury (including common assault), be it the actual committing of an act or a wilful reckless attempt; (ii) other aggressive behaviour where the staff member has reason to believe that the perpetrator, through physical contact, will inflict pain and or injury (including common assault) to him/herself or another intentionally or recklessly.
>
> (*Hampshire Social Services, 1991b*)

The social work profession has begun to address the issue. In the future, many more authorities will be pressed into releasing scarce training resources in an attempt to encourage and develop the use of professional control and restraint techniques. The Home Office acknowledge that the techniques have been taught to and are used by organizations, such as the social services (Home Office, 1991).

Some critics of training in the use of physical restraint techniques argue that it leads to the use of control and restraint as the primary means of coping with the potentially violent client. However, Gilbert (1988) suggests that:

> Staff who have completed the course gain in confidence and this is reflected in their work. It has been observed that, because of this increased confidence, they are likely to initiate a physical response to a difficult situation later than those who have not been trained; this clearly gives more chance for a counselling approach to succeed.

> *(Gilbert, 1988)*

Counselling

Rowett, commenting on his experience when interviewing those who had been assaulted, said that it was not uncommon for those who had been attacked to break down and weep. Indeed, Halliley wrote (Halliley, 1986), 'They had not told anyone of the attack, or attacks; they had bottled it up for years. In some instances, the research interview became a therapeutic interview'.

Hampshire Social Services identified the need for a professional counselling service for victims of assault or the threat of such (Clark and Kidd, 1990). Birmingham Social Services, following the death of Frances Bettridge, made counselling support available from a specially appointed member of staff.

Hampshire's provision for counselling victims of violence was very successful from the moment the scheme started (Hampshire Social Services, 1991a). Several part-time counsellors were recruited from the social services and probation departments. In return for an annual honorarium, counsellors are available to provide a service to victims who request such following an approach to the co-ordinator of the service. One of the important roles of the co-ordinator (who is employed by the social services department as a psychologist) is to listen carefully to what the victim says, identify the needs of the member of staff, and then select carefully the most appropriate counsellor to work with the individual. The service supported 185 people in the period December 1989 to June 1991. In September 1991, 12 to 15 people a month were being supported.

The arrangement whereby it is possible for a counsellor to be selected from outside the victim's own department appears to be very satisfactory in terms of providing full support while, at the same time, retaining utmost confidentiality for the person being counselled. There is the added advantage of greater flexibility in being able to select from a wide range of counselling skills. This is invaluable when matching a prospective counsellor with a victim. These factors would appear to go some way towards answering Norris' plea for an independent violence agency (Norris, 1990). Norris makes the relevant point that:

> A counselling service, genuinely independent of a social worker's managers or work associates, could facilitate accurate feedback because the anonymity of those who have suffered can be assured.
>
> *(Norris, 1990)*

It would be helpful to explore this issue with social workers who have been involved in a counselling process. More importantly, perhaps, it should be explored with staff members who, because of their concern about confidentiality, as well as the frequently irrational feelings of guilt experienced by victims, have thought twice about approaching their 'in-house' counselling service despite the proffered assurances.

Doctors have their own, independent and voluntary counselling service (*British Medical Journal*, 1988). Interestingly, despite its independence, strict confidentiality has also made this service difficult to evaluate. Any doctor, colleague or spouse can telephone a London number and be put in touch with an advisor in the same speciality as the doctor in need of help, but not resident in the same locality. So Norris' suggestion of a similar agency for social workers may not be so extreme as first impressions would seem to suggest.

There do not appear to be any studies that have taken account of threats made against relatives or friends of the social work victim. In a situation where the aggressive client confronts the social worker with 'I know where your kids go to school . . . ' one wonders whether and to what extent the employer should provide counselling, or even protection, for members of the social worker's family. On the grounds that severe and realistic threats to family will inevitably have a detrimental effect upon work performance, any money invested in family support could certainly be money well spent. In Australia it would seem that the need for supportive intervention has been acknowledged and provided for family and friends of bank hold-up victims (Bowie, 1989).

Compensation and prosecution

Even in the best departments where thought has been given to the arrangements to protect staff and prevent violence, the occasional incident will arise and the social worker will experience financial loss in addition to physical pain and injury. All local authorities and health authorities have insurance schemes that usually provide cover for employees who are injured while carrying out their professional responsibilities. Larger authorities sometimes cover their own risks. It remains incumbent upon employees to ascertain the extent of cover. It should never be necessary for individuals to take out additional personal insurance.

Hampshire Social Services have taken seriously their responsibility to try to ensure that assaulted staff are fully supported. In the first 6 months of the financial year 1991/1992 £6000 was spent on ex-gratia payments to staff suffering damage to possessions, including vehicles, and payment of the first £250 of legal fees in respect of independent advice.

In addition to the employers' insurance arrangements, victims of assault will want to consider the option of seeking compensation from the assailant through proceedings in the civil court. It is also possible to ask for compensation in the criminal court following a successful police or private prosecution. The final recourse is to apply for compensation from the Criminal Injuries Compensation Board if all the appropriate conditions are met (Chapter 7). While many authorities are careful not to advise any one course of action, it is reasonable to expect a post-incident counsellor to outline the options so that the assaulted person can decide the most appropriate course of action. Traditionally, social workers have felt guilty about taking a client to court. They have been reluctant to take this course of action. The pendulum has swung and many now see it for what it is – a legitimate tool to assist in curbing the aggressor's enthusiasm.

SUMMARY

A considerable amount of work has been done during the past few years in an attempt to increase our knowledge and expertise so that violence by clients can be anticipated and prevented. It has been acknowledged consistently that, in several situations and sometimes for inexplicable reasons, something will trigger a violent response and, regardless of training and professional ability, a social worker will be seriously injured. In a few cases people will continue to die.

Nevertheless, things must be learnt from this experience and from the advice and expertise of those who have given time and effort to try to ensure that all colleagues who died did not die in vain. Health and safety legislation clearly gives responsibility to employees as well as employers. There must be no attempt by anyone to opt out in the hope that all will be well. Research referred to in this chapter makes reference to an attitude by some social workers that can, at best, be described as cavalier. Others would label it reckless. In other areas of responsibility, social workers have demonstrated their ability to be thoroughly professional and caring. This applies, particularly, in situations where support has been necessary for colleagues who have been assaulted. Sadly, it seems that in many cases, it has been necessary for them to assume the supportive role because line managers have not provided a satisfactory response.

The Nova study (Norris, 1990) suggests that some people believe that a greater proportion of social workers are reporting incidents of violence. Hopefully, that is a correct assumption. Senior managers should make it easy for staff to make reports. Some standardization of documentation will undoubtedly facilitate the collation of information that will, in turn, enable better conclusions to be drawn and more lessons learnt. While senior managers must take responsibility for devising meaningful documentation, professional organizations and trade unions should take the initiative in ensuring the introduction of a standardized process. Working together for the care and protection of our staff members is everybody's responsibility. Only a concerted effort will reduce the level of risk to acceptable proportions.

REFERENCES

Association of Directors of Social Services (1987) *Guidelines and Recommendations to Employers on Violence Against Employees*, ADSS, London.

Barnett, P. (1985) Letter to *The Guardian*, 6 April 1985.

Bowie, V. (1989) *Coping with Violence: A Guide for the Human Services*, Karibuni Press, New South Wales, Australia.

British Association of Social Workers (1988) *Violence to Social Workers*, BASW, Birmingham.

British Medical Journal (1988) Scrutator, *BMJ*, **297**, 3.

Brown, R.A., Bute, S.F., and Ford, P.K. (1986) *Social Workers at Risk: The Prevention and Management of Violence*, Macmillan, London.

Bute, S.F. (1979a) An indictment upon us for failing to learn. *Social Work Today*, 6 February.

Bute, S.F. (1979b) The threat of violence in close encounters with clients. *Social Work Today*, 4 December.

Bute, S.F. (1980) *Staff Guidelines on the Management of Violence*, Hampshire Social Services, Southampton.

Clark, S. and Kidd, B. (1990) Part of the job. *Social Work Today*, 19 July.

Department of Health and Social Security (1976) The management of violent, or potentially violent, hospital patients. *Health Circular* (76) 11 March.

Department of Health and Social Security (1988) *Report of the Committee of*

Inquiry into the Care and Aftercare of Miss Sharon Campbell, HMSO, London.

Dooley, E. (1988) The management of potentially dangerous patients in the community. *Bulletin of the Royal College of Psychiatrists*, **12**, 419–21.

Gilbert, J. (1988) Exercising some restraint. *Social Work Today*, **20**(8), 16–18.

Halliley, M. (1986) The Burden of the Social Workers' Guilty Secret. *The Guardian*, 16 April 1986.

Hampshire Social Services (1990) *Report to Departmental Management Team*, Hampshire County Council, Winchester.

Hampshire Social Services (1991a) *Report to Chief Officers' Management Group*, Hampshire County Council, Winchester.

Hampshire Social Services (1991b) *Using Physical Restraint: Practice Guidance for Social Services Staff*, Hampshire County Council, Winchester.

Hansard (1986) House of Commons – The Parliamentary Debates 29.4.1986, p. 395.

Health and Safety Executive (1991) *Health and Safety Information Bulletin* **186**, HSE, London.

Health Services Advisory Committee (1987) *Violence to Staff in the Health Services*, HMSO, London.

Home Office (1991) Guidelines on control and restraint, in *Using Physical Restraint: Practice Guidance for Social Services Staff*, Hampshire County Council, Winchester.

Hudson, B. (1990) Loking for a way out. *Health Service Journal*, **100**(818), 1354–55.

Johnson, S. (1987) *Guidelines for Social Workers in Coping with Violent Clients: an Analysis of Selected Guidelines*. Unpublished dissertation, University of Southampton.

Jones, D. (1986) *The Personal Social Services Perspective*. Unpublished report of DHSS conference on *Violence to Staff*, London, 2 December 1986.

Kedward, C. (1990) *University of Sussex National Research Study in Violence against Social Workers (D. Norris)*, Jessica Kingsley, London, pp. 62–124.

Norris, D. (1990) *Violence against Social Workers: The Implications for Practice*, Jessica Kingsley, London.

Phillips, R. and Leadbetter, D. (1990) Violent sessions in the classroom. *Social Work Today*, **21**(21), 22–23.

Poyner, B. and Warne, C. (1986) *Violence to Staff: A Basis for Assessment and Prevention*, Health and Safety Executive, HMSO, London.

Rowett, C. (1986) *Violence in Social Work*, University of Cambridge Institute of Criminology, Cambridge.

Saunders, L. (1987) *Safe and Secure in Surrey?* Violence to staff of the Social Services Department, Social Services Research, University of Birmingham Department of Social Policy and Social Work, Birmingham, Nos. 5/6, pp.32–55.

Stockdale, J. and Phillips, C. (1991) *Violence at Work: Issues, Policies and Procedures – A Case Study of Two Local Authorities*, Local Government Management Board, Luton.

Strathclyde Regional Council (1987) *Violence to Staff: Policies and Procedures*, Strathclyde Regional Council Social Work Department, Strathclyde.

Surrey County Council (1987) *Safe and Secure in Surrey?* Report of the Social

Services Working Group on *Violence to Staff*, Social Services Department, Surrey.

Townsend, D. (1985) Letter to *The Guardian*, 1 May 1985.

CHAPTER 4

Aggression towards general practitioners

F.D. Richard Hobbs

INTRODUCTION

Most general practitioners (GPs) will experience, at some stage during their professional lives, concerns for their safety at work. For some doctors, these fears will be a regular and perhaps even an expected feature of the job. For others, events that involve aggression will be infrequent and totally unexpected. Little is accurately known about GP experiences of violence or how it affects the practitioner. Much of this chapter is therefore devoted to the results of a major survey into aggression in general practice carried out in 1989. This study not only provides us with a snapshot of the scale of the problem but, perhaps more importantly, helps to identify some of the factors that precipitate violence in the community and thereby offers the potential for avoidance of the risk.

What little published work on aggression in general practice that does exist has been based either on small surveys (Neville, 1986; D'Urso and Hobbs, 1989; Walls, 1983) or on anecdotal personal reports (Savage, 1984; Cambrowicz *et al.*, 1987; Raghu, 1979; Siriwardene, 1987; Anonymous, 1978). Evidence about the consequences for the victim and about the general level of intimidation experienced by doctors is even less well documented (Harris, 1989). Various factors may lead doctors to avoid discussing or reporting that they have suffered abuse (Council of Family Practitioners Committees, 1987). It might be seen as an inevitable feature of the job (D'Urso and Hobbs, 1989). Suffering regular abuse may even be seen as a consequence of poor doctoring skills (Fricker, 1987). Anonymity is sometimes sought because victims fear retribution (Anonymous, 1988). Indeed there may be concern to avoid publicity in case this presents general practitioners as 'legitimate' targets. This lack of information on aggression towards general practitioners contrasts badly with the data available on violence to other groups in close contact with the public, such as teachers (National Association of School Masters/Union of Women Teachers, 1986), social workers (Brown *et al.*, 1986; Strathclyde Regional Council Social Work Department, 1986), transport workers (Department of Transport, 1986; Rose, 1976), and community nurses (Department of Health and Social Security, 1987). The lesson one should learn from the studies in other disciplines is that the results of survey can be used to develop preventative strategies (Brown *et al.*, 1986; Strathclyde Regional Council Social Work Department, 1986; Department of Transport, 1986; Iliffe and Hang, 1991).

THE GENERAL PRACTITIONER SURVEY

The principal aim of the 1989 GP study was to survey the extent of abuse and violence directed towards a large sample of general practitioners during the course of their professional duties. Previous studies had identified some of the precipitants of violence (Rasheeduddin, 1981, which include alcohol (D'Urso and Hobbs, 1989), drug abuse, and mental illness (Short, 1981; Woolf 1982), but little else of note. A second aim was, therefore, to categorize the severity, frequency, location and precipitants of this reported aggression. The final aim was to explore the feelings of intimidation experienced by practitioners who had suffered abuse and note whether aggression had stimulated changes to practice (Hobbs, 1991).

Who was interviewed?

A questionnaire, piloted in an earlier small survey, was posted to all unrestricted principals in contract with the Family Practitioner Committees of the West Midlands Regional Health Authority in March 1989 – a total of 2694 doctors. A short covering letter explaining the purpose of the study was included with an addressed but not stamped envelope for the reply. The questionnaire consisted of predominantly closed questions, with tables to record incidents of aggression with the scale of violence on one axis and characteristics on the other. Open questions elicited the views of the doctors on violence in practice. The practitioners worked in a wide variety of practices, from those in deprived, inner-city locations to those in rural communities.

Confidential details were obtained on the age and sex of the doctor, medical school of qualification, number of partners and practice location. A scale was devised, which categorized aggression into five degrees of increasing severity:

I = verbal abuse;

II = verbal abuse with specific threats (e.g. shaking fist) or with physical action against inanimate objects (e.g. banging table, throwing object, forcing a door);

III = physical action against the person without injury (e.g. pushing or obstructing);

IV = physical violence with minor injury (e.g. cuts, bruises); and

V = physical violence with severe injury (e.g. knocked out, needing hospital care).

Except for the addition of category II in this study, the scale was similar to that used in the largest published survey on violence in the health service (Health Services Advisory Committee, 1987). This earlier study investigated the recollections of 3000 workers in a variety of grades and roles within the hospital and community services.

Practitioners were requested to recall the frequency of aggressive episodes in the previous 12 months, providing details on the level of aggression, the location of the incident, the age and health status of the aggressor, and the main precipitation factor. Doctors were also questioned on their level of concern over aggression, during various periods of the working day and at night. A list of any changes made to the practice due to aggression were recorded. Finally, details were requested on the frequency of aggression towards receptionists and other staff.

Who replied?

Of the 2694 unrestricted principals, 1093 returned their questionnaire, representing a 41% response. Although this was a low percentage response, the characteristics of the responders to national averages were similar for age and sex of the doctor and size of practice, as can be seen in Table 4.1. The only highly significant difference was an under-representation of GPs who had qualified outside the United Kingdom and a slightly significant lack of doctors over 65, within the responding sample.

Inevitably, the low response will have reduced the study's ability to provide an objective survey on violence towards family doctors. Furthermore, relying on recollections of incidents (as have all previous studies) rather than prospective recording further erodes objectivity. However, the study accurately represents the perceptions of responding practitioners to their personal level of violence and it remains a powerful survey of their views. Although the percentage response to the questionnaire was low, the actual number of replies was

Table 4.1 Characteristics of the sample population compared with national estimates

Characteristic	Sample [a] (n = 1093)	National figures [b]
Age of the GP (years)		
<35	215 (19.8)	208 (19.1)
35–44	398 (36.7)	335 (30.7)
45–54	270 (24.9)	270 (24.8)
55–64	177 (16.3)	227 (20.8)
65>	24 (2.2)	50 (4.6)
Where GP was qualified		
Britain	921 (84.3)	18 394 (73.8)
India, Pakistan	109 (10.0)	⎫
Other	29 (2.7)	⎬ 6528 (26.2)
Not known	34 (3.1)	⎭
Sex of the GP		
Male	900 (82.3)	900 (82.6)
Female	190 (17.4)	190 (17.4)
Not known	3 (0.3)	– –
Number of partners in practice		
Single	121 (11.1)	3007 (11.3)
2–3	369 (33.8)	9309 (35.1)
4–5	43 (36.8)	8950 (33.7)
6+	200 (18.3)	5243 (19.8)

[a] Figures are no. (%) of practitioners.
[b] National percentages derived from DHSS (1989) for age and sex (n = 1090), DOH (1989) for where qualified (n = 24 922) and OHE (1987) for partnership size (n = 26 509).

huge and the study provides the largest recorded database on aggression directed at professional health service staff. It represented the experiences of nearly 4% of all general practitioners in England and Wales.

The main concern that the low response poses is that general practitioners suffering aggression were more motivated to reply and are therefore over-represented in the sample. However, the 119 responders (11% of the sample) who had experienced assault or injury in the previous year, produced a similar rate to previous surveys, which reported 11% (Harris, 1989), 10% (Neville, 1986) and 11% (D'Urso and Hobbs, 1989). Furthermore, 405 doctors (37%) in the sample had not suffered any sort of abuse in the previous year. This figure compares with only 9% who had not suffered abuse in a previous (urban) GP survey (D'Urso and Hobbs, 1989).

Who suffers from violence?

Of the 1093 responders, 687 (63%) had suffered some form of aggression in the previous year, with 100 (15%) of these stating that it was increasing and 31 (5%) that it was decreasing. Figure 4.1 shows that 157 (14%) of the responding practitioners suffered regular verbal abuse (at least once a month), with 31 (3%) experiencing regular threatening behaviour and three (0.3%) regular minor assault or obstruction. In the group of doctors who had actually suffered aggression during the 12 months, these percentages rose to 23%, 5% and 0.4% respectively. Of the sample, 1% had to tolerate verbal abuse every day. Thirty-six GPs (3%) had received minor injuries from an assault in the previous year and five doctors (0.4%) had suffered a severe injury.

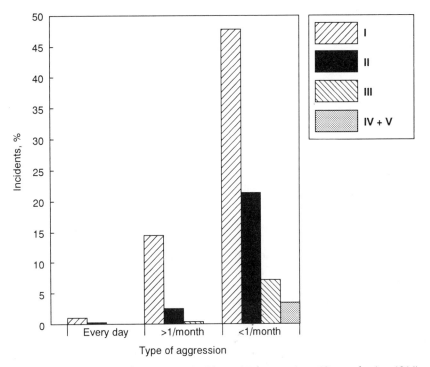

Figure 4.1 Frequency of aggressive incidents in the previous 12 months (*n* = 1014).

Where does violence occur?

The majority (57%) of the 1664 incidents displayed in Figure 4.2 occurred in the surgery, with 669 (40%) of all events described as taking place in the consulting room. Some 1520 (91%) of the events exclusively involved some level of verbal abuse; however, 41 (3%) involved actual injury. Serious violence happened more on domiciliary

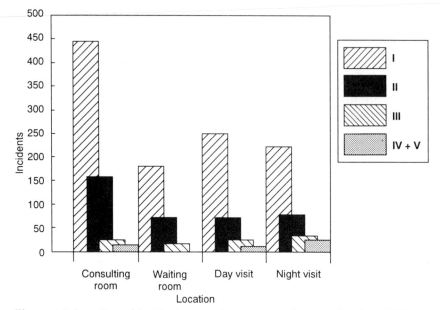

Figure 4.2 Location of incidents according to type of aggression ($n = 1776$).

visits, particularly at night, with doctors indicating that 24 (23%) assaults and 8 (22%) actual injuries had occurred on day visits and 36 (35%) assaults and 22 (53%) actual injuries on night visits.

Who is aggressive?

As in previous surveys, the usual instigators of aggression turned out to be men, numbering 1166 (66%) of all cases as shown in Figure 4.3. Of these, 664 (37%) were described as male patients and a surprisingly high figure of 441 (25%) as male relatives. Indeed, a total of 668 (38) of the aggressors were denoted as being relatives of patients. Of obstructions, assaults and injuries, 76% were attributed to men. Aggression was almost exclusively associated with direct patient contact since only 5% of incidents involved the general public, 90% of such events involving verbal abuse only.

In most incidents, the aggressor (Figure 4.4) was under 40 years of age (76% of cases). There was no difference between the 15–29 and 30–39 age bands. This 3:1 age preponderance of under 40-year-olds was consistent, whatever the type of aggression that occurred. This rather surprising finding that it is not predominantly the young who engage in aggression towards general practitioners concurs with another smaller study where the average age of the aggressor was 40 years (Neville, 1986).

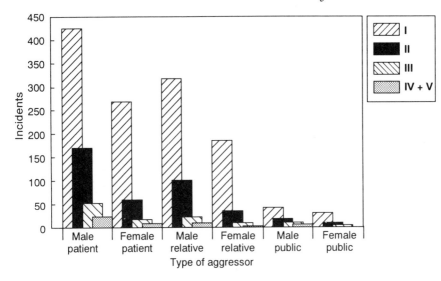

Figure 4.3 Type of aggressor according to type of aggression (*n* = 1776).

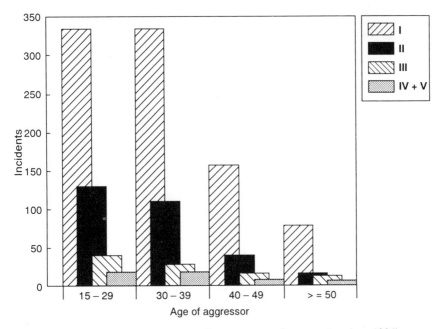

Figure 4.4 Age of aggressor according to type of aggression (n = 1334).

What are the precipitants?

Factors most frequently reported as precipitating aggression were drugs or alcohol in 464 (27%) cases and anxiety in 435 (26%) cases, as seen in Figure 4.5. Interestingly, the most commonly quoted cause for verbal abuse (29% of responders) was an anxious patient, a factor not noted in any previous study. Anxiety was the second most common cause (22% of responders) of threatening verbal abuse and was even implicated in 11% of assaults. Two additional factors that could be associated with anxiety, a long wait for patients and a recent bereavement, were reported 183 (11%) and 86 (5%) times respectively. Virtually all of these latter precipitants (261 out of the 269 responses) were confined to some type of verbal abuse.

Mental illness was only implicated in 258 responses (15%) that noted abuse. However, this factor became the most important one for serious incidents involving assault or injury. In these incidents, it was recorded by 56 out of 147 (38%) responders, closely followed by alcohol or drugs with 54 (37%) responses.

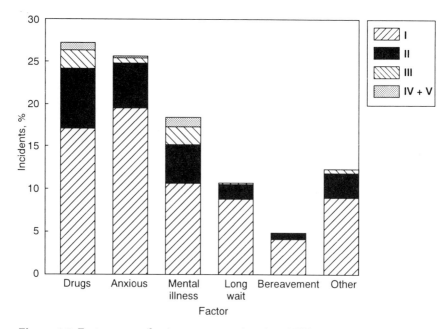

Figure 4.5 Factors contributing to aggression ($n = 1692$).

Have doctors changed their practice?

Altogether, some 299 (27%) of the responding doctors had made changes to their practice directly because of aggression (Hobbs, 1994a). The commonest changes included striking more patients off their list

(12%); installing panic buttons (9%); using the deputizing service more (7%); installing protective screens in reception (6%); or calling the police more to surgery or on visits (5% and 3%). However, more personal changes included feeling less committed to medicine (7%); feeling less confident (4%); prescribing on demand to angry patients (4%); and even refusing to visit in certain areas (2%).

The survey further revealed (Table 4.2) that doctors who had suffered abuse were continuing to feel stressed about aggression (Hobbs, 1994b). A massive 74% of them felt some degree of intimidation on night calls (between 11.00p.m. and 7.00a.m.): for 20% this was described as severe at times and 6% were always fearful on night visits. The respective figures for evening calls (7.00–11.00p.m.) were 72%, 13% and 3%.

Table 4.2 Survey of doctors ($n = 687$) who had suffered abuse: place of consultation and feelings of intimidation

Feelings of intimidation	Doctor activity (% of responders)				
	Consulting in surgery $n = 611$	On call at home $n = 507$	Visits in day $n = 512$	Visits 7.00– 11.00p.m. $n = 565$	Visits after 11.00p.m. $n = 565$
Never	254 (42)	290 (57)	280 (55)	156 (28)	146 (26)
Occasional mild	304 (50)	182 (36)	212 (41)	316 (56)	286 (51)
Occasional, severe	36 (6)	22 (4)	14 (3)	50 (9)	71 (13)
Frequent, mild	9 (2)	6 (1)	2 (0.4)	17 (3)	23 (4)
Frequent, severe	4 (1)	3 (1)	2 (0.4)	11 (2)	8 (1)
Always fearful	4 (1)	4 (1)	2 (0.4)	15 (3)	31 (6)

Summary

This survey confirmed that aggression during the working day is a regular feature for many general practitioners. Some 687 (63%) of those replying had suffered aggression during the previous 12 months, 191 (18%) had experienced some type of abuse at least once per month, with 11 (1%) being verbally abused every day. Even if all the nonresponders were assumed to have avoided any abuse, then at least 26% of general practitioners had experienced violence at work. Extrapolating the 1664 events over the year to the total 2694 doctors surveyed and assuming that the nonresponders experience no aggression would produce a minimum incidence of aggression in general practice of 0.62 events per doctor year (1.52 events per responding

GP per year or 2.42 events per year among those GPs who have suffered abuse). It was worrying to note that of those doctors who experienced aggression, over 14% felt it was increasing. Although aggression is common, it seems confined to certain groups of doctors, since nearly 40% of responders in this sample never suffered any abuse from patients.

Most incidents involved verbal abuse alone but the effects of this are difficult to predict accurately. Where this abuse is persistent (in 1% of the sample it occurred every day) it is likely to have a detrimental effect on doctors (Harris, 1989), their staff (Health Services Advisory Committee, 1987) and indeed other waiting patients. It would also be interesting to note how many of the incidents of assault or injury had escalated from simple verbal abuse.

Some 942 (57%) events took place in the surgery, but more serious incidents of violence (58% of assaults and 75% of injuries) were more likely to occur on visits, especially at night. This study confirmed that being a male (66% of cases), the influence of alcohol or drugs (27%) and mental illness (19%) were frequent precipitants of abuse – particularly the more serious forms. New findings were the frequent involvement of relatives in aggression with 668 (38%) cases and the major precipitants of anxiety or the experience of a long wait by the aggressor in 435 (26%) and 183 (11%) events, respectively. Such contributory factors are worth monitoring by doctors and their staff since early recognition and careful intervention may prevent subsequent actions of aggression.

There should be concern for the well-being of the 7% of general practitioners frequently or always very fearful when on night visits. This extreme level of intimidation was also experienced by 5% of doctors when performing evening visits and 1% during surgery consultations. It is therefore unexpected that changes in personal feelings towards medicine were volunteered, with some feeling less committed to medicine, others less confident and a few thinking of giving up practice because of fears over aggression. Such feelings indicate the low morale among general practitioners, although these findings were not so depressing as the 30% of 120 inner-city doctors in another study who indicated they would not continue general practice/medicine (Myerson, 1991).

Some of the understandable coping strategies employed by the doctors could exacerbate the problem of aggression. Examples of these are:

- prescribing on demand, which might induce an influx of addicts;
- increasing the use of deputizing services, which probably increases out-of-hours calls;
- installing protective screens, which have been shown to increase

- violent incidents (Council of Family Practitioners Committees, 1987); and
- striking off aggressive patients as this simply transfers the problem.

Some sensible, although involved, strategies such as taking someone else on visits (especially employed by women doctors) could be interpreted as significantly increasing the actual and human cost of providing an out-of-hours health service. For 2% of doctors, the price of night visits was obviously too high and they refused to visit certain areas. Such an action is potentially a breach of the doctor's terms of service and could place patients in that area at some risk.

Perhaps the time has come to reconsider seriously the requirement for all general practitioners to provide continuous 24 hour cover to all their patients. This issue is being debated increasingly (Iliffe and Hang, 1991; Bolam *et al.*, 1988) and was raised in the GMSC discussion document, *Building Your own Future* (General Medical Services Committee, 1991). It touched such a nerve among GPs that many local medical committees (LMCs) raised the issue at the 1992 national LMC representatives conference, where the motion was passed to seek an end to the 24 hour contractual commitment for GPs. This will now form the basis of future negotiations with the Department of Health. Out-of-hours visits may represent only 4% of consultations in general practice (Wilkin *et al.*, 1987), but 74% of doctors in this sample expressed some degree of fear over aggression on night calls.

The Department of Health should be concerned for the health of their contractors and could consider experimenting with alternative strategies, such as an FHSA-organized night-visit service with escorts for the doctors. Perhaps out-of-hours medical services should become an FHSA rather than practice responsibility? It might also seem reasonable to expect FHSA flexibility over the 26 hour per week doctor/patient contact time for those doing especially stressful out-of-hours cover (i.e. time off in the day in lieu of out-of-hours visits).

Studying the causes and effects of aggression towards health service staff remains important. The risks to non health service staff such as social workers or housing office staff have generated sufficient concern among employers to fund experiments in safer ways of providing services. Examples of change in their practice include the provision of two-way radios to social workers and enabling joint visiting in many circumstances. Local housing departments have researched better office environments (Health and Safety Executive, 1988) where the public contact the service directly (using open-plan rooms, carpets, better fabrics, plants and soft lighting) and providing specific training in interpersonal skills. Such initiatives require investment by the service providers. The returns on such investment are improved confidence and effectiveness of staff (Health and Safety

Executive, 1988), reduced staff turnover (Poyner and Warne, 1986) and reduced levels of aggression from members of the public (Health and Safety Executive, 1988).

The self-employed status of general practice militates against such major initiatives but, on a practical note, general practitioners should heed some of the lessons learnt by others. Furthermore, there are legal responsibilities for GPs as employers to provide acceptable and safe working environments for their staff, who may also suffer aggression from patients. This should include the addition of assault cover on surgery insurance.

FORMULATING A PRACTICE PROTOCOL

GPs who suffer aggression must talk about it within their practice and with colleagues. Aggression is more likely to occur when working with certain patient groups: (i) the drunk or drug-influenced; (ii) the disturbed and agitated; (iii) anxious patients; or (iv) those who have had to wait a long time. The practice should have set protocols for dealing with such groups. Such protocols should include details on what staff should do:

- to predict what might trigger anger from a patient;
- if surgeries are running late (such as to announce why to the waiting room or offer an alternative and early appointment);
- if a patient shouts;
- when deciding when to call the police;
- when deciding what follow-up should occur for the abused staff and the aggressor patient.

Ideally these should have been agreed at staff meetings, where everyone has the opportunity for personal input. Staff should already receive training in interpersonal skills to be effective in their numerous roles. Such skills become absolutely essential when handling abusive patients. One programme for training practice managers and GPs to formulate a practice protocol has been produced (Harris et al., 1993).

The doctor should accept responsibility for handling aggression where and as soon as it occurs, interrupting consulting if necessary. This will not only support staff but also allow the patient's concerns to be addressed promptly and may possibly avoid escalation. A quick response is likely to be a positive sign to the two-fifths of patients who become aggressive owing to anxiety or because they have been kept waiting.

A further responsibility for the doctor is to discuss the episode with the patients at a later and hopefully calmer occasion. This should preferably be an invitation to attend an appointment rather than a letter discussing the incident. It is then possible to probe gently for the reasons why the incident occurred so that desirable changes to practice can be identified and discussed with the patient. However, the display of aggression at the surgery is not acceptable and the patient must understand this. Persistent or serious offenders may need to be removed from the list. Assault or injury should always be reported to the police and compensation be sought from the offender or Criminal Injuries Board (Chapter 8)

For any health issue, the main priority for the practice must be attention to the prevention of aggression. The surgery environment should be regularly reviewed. Open-plan, deep reception counters would seem the ideal, perhaps with a slightly raised platform on the receptionist's side (Health and Safety Executive, 1988). Waiting room seating should be soft and there should be sufficient space to avoid crowding (Health and Safety Executive, 1988). Soft toys (avoiding noisy ones) and reading material should be provided. Lighting should be adequate but soft, avoiding fluorescent strips (Health and Safety Executive, 1988). Consulting rooms should be similarly attractive and sound-proofed. Staff should be trained in the early recognition of the signs of a patient who is becoming agitated.

Such attention to surgery decor and layout has major implications for the uptake of cost rent schemes and improvement grants. Family Health Service Authorities should give very serious support to practices that suffer regular aggression and should consider maximizing improvement grants on improvements directed towards safer surgeries.

The risk of aggression is a further major impetus to doctors (and medical students) to develop good communication skills. Particular emphasis in teaching such skills should be directed to the handling of these patients who are disinhibited, whether through mental illness or chemical abuse. Scenarios involving escalating levels of abuse in differing consultations would be excellent material for role-play sessions at medical schools.

Two of the lynchpins of general practice, its accessibility and the intimacy of the consultation, will inevitably increase the vulnerability of general practitioners to abuse. It seems likely that the experience of aggression, or even the fear of it, will undermine the confidence of doctors. How much this serves to erode the quality of the doctor–patient relationship, the availability of services and the dedication of staff is an important question that remains to be answered.

REFERENCES

Anonymous (1978) Assaults on doctors. *British Medical Journal*, **1**, 1229–30.

Anonymous (1988) Fear keeps GPs silent. *Pulse*, **48**, 12.

Bolam, M., McCartney, M., and Modell, M. (1988) Patients' assessment of out-of-hours care in general practice. *British Medical Journal*, **296**, 829–32.

Brown, R., Bute, S., and Ford, P. (1986) *Social Workers at Risk: The Prevention and Management of Violence*, Macmillan, London.

Cambrowicz, S., Ford, P.G.T., Winn, J.C. *et al.* (1987) Assault on a GP. *British Medical Journal*, **294**, 616–18.

Council of Family Practitioners Committees (1987) Attacks and robberies involving doctors. *Family Practitioner Services*, **14**, 278–79.

Department of Health (1989) *Health and Personal Social Service Statistics for England*, HMSO, London.

Department of Health and Social Security (1987) *General Medical Practitioners' Workloads*, HMSO, London.

Department of Health and Social Security (1989) *Violence to Staff: Report of DHSS Advisory Committee on Violence to Staff*, HMSO, London.

Department of Transport (1986) *Assaults on Bus Staff and Measures to Prevent Such Assaults: Report on the Working Group on Violence to Road Passenger Transport Staff*, HMSO, London.

D'Urso, P. and Hobbs, F.D.R. (1989) Aggression and the general practitioner. *British Medical Journal*, **298**, 97–8.

Fricker, J. (1987) So you think you're safe? *Journal of Royal College of General Practitioners*, **37**, 426–27.

General Medical Services Committee. (1991) *Building Your Own Future: An Agenda for General Practice*, Tavistock, London.

Harris, A. (1989) Violence in general practice. *British Medical Journal*, **293**, 63–64.

Harris, A., Wykes, T., Brisby, T. *et al* (1993) *The Prevention of Violence in General Practice: A Training Manual*, Lambeth, Southwark & Lewisham FHSA, London.

Health and Safety Executive (1988) *Preventing Violence to Staff*, HMSO, London.

Health Services Advisory Committee (1987) *Violence to Staff in the Health Services*, HMSO, London.

Hobbs, F.D.R. (1991) Violence in general practice: a survey of general practitioners' views. *British Medical Journal*, **302**, 329–32.

Hobbs, F.D.R. (1994a) General practitioners' changes to practice due to aggression at work. *Family Practice*, in press.

Hobbs, F.D.R. (1994b) Fear of aggression at work in general practitioners who have suffered serious episodes of abuse. *British Journal of General Practice*, in press.

Iliffe, S. and Hang, U. (1991) Out of hours work in general practice. *British Medical Journal*, **302**, 1584–86.

Myerson, S. (1991) Violence to general practitioners and fear of violence. *Family Practice*, **8**, 145–47.

National Association of School Masters/Union of Women Teachers (1986) *Pupil Violence and Serious Disorder in Schools*, NASUWT, Birmingham.

Neville, R.G. (1986) Violent patients in general practice. *Practitioner*, **230**, 1105–8.

Office of Health Economics (1987) *Compendium of Health Statistics*. 6th edn, HMSO, London.

Poyner, B. and Warne, C. (1986) *Violence to Staff: A Basis for Assessment and Prevention*, HMSO, London.

Raghu, K. (1979) Aggressive patients – what is the answer? *British Medical Journal*, **2**, 1147.

Rasheeduddin, K. (1981) Violence and socioeconomic development, in *Violence and its Causes*, (eds J.M. Domenach *et al.*), Unesco, Paris, pp. 167–85.

Rose, J.S. (1976) *A Study of Violence on London Transport*, Behavioral Science Unit, Establishments Department, Greater London Council, London.

Savage, R. (1984) Violence. *British Medical Journal*, **289**, 1618–19.

Short, P.W. (1981) The psychiatrically violent patient. *British Medical Journal*, **282**, 281–28.

Siriwardene, S.K. (1987) Doctor at risk. *Physician*, **6**, 333.

Strathclyde Regional Council Social Work Department (1986) *Violence to Staff: Policies and Procedures*, Strathclyde Council/NALGO, Strathclyde and London.

Walls, F. (1983) Assault. *British Medical Journal*, **286**, 113–14.

Wilkin, D., Hallam, L., Leavey, R. *et al.* (1987) *Anatomy of Urban General Practice*. Tavistock Publications, London.

Woolf, P.G. (1982) Subnormality and violence. *Practitioner*, **226**, 503–4.

CHAPTER 5

Sexual victimization in the workplace

Gillian Mezey

INTRODUCTION

While physical violence can be regarded as an occupational hazard for professionals who work with individuals who are unpredictable, mentally disturbed or simply opportunistic, sexual violence in the form of harassment or intimidation represents a risk for patients and staff alike. Both health professionals and patients are vulnerable to all forms of sexual exploitation and abuse, including harassment, indecent assault and rape. The perpetrators may be colleagues, clients or patients and it may take place in any of the varied settings that health professionals operate in.

While certain violent sexual assaults, including rape, are recognized and commonly dealt with as criminal acts, other sexually intimidating behaviours represent victimization of a subtle and pernicious kind and may not be recognized for what they are. Certain factors may also serve to neutralize and minimize the significance of any sexual encounter within health care facilities, for example, the attempted rape of a mentally ill inpatient may be dismissed on the basis that she or he does not understand what is happening or is less likely to be affected by it. The molestation of a female staff nurse by her supervisor who 'accidentally' touches her breasts may be rationalized as friendliness. There is a reluctance for both patients and health professionals to recognize that hospitals are anything but safe havens and that, once identified as a carer or someone to be cared for, the individual's sexuality, sexual impulses and sexual fantasies are denied. This is particularly curious given the still popular stereotypes of nurses either as sexually available and promiscuous or as virginal, altruistic, 'angels'. Sexual victimization represents an assault on the dignity and integrity of the victim and undermines assumptions about safety and competency, even in the absence of overt violence or physical injury.

This chapter will discuss two forms of sexual victimization that have a particular impact for the practice and security of health professionals and the safety of their patients: (i) sexual harassment; and (ii) therapist–patient sexual contact.

LEGISLATION

Relevant legislation pertaining to the sexual abuse or assault on patients, clients or staff is summarized as follows:

1. *Health and Safety at Work Act 1974*
   Provision for the reasonable safety of employees at work is a legal obligation.
2. *S1 (1) Sex Discrimination Act 1975*
   A person discriminates against a woman in any circumstance . . . if on the grounds of her sex he treats her less favourably than he . . . would treat a man.
3. *S41 (1) Sex Discrimination Act 1975*
   This sets out the principle of employer liability and makes an employer legally responsible for any offence committed by one of his employees in the course of carrying out his normal work activities unless it can be shown under S41 (3) that he took steps as were reasonably practical to prevent his doing that act.
4. *Sexual Offences (Amendment) Act 1976*
   A man commits rape if he has unlawful sexual intercourse with a woman when (a) she does not consent to it, (b) he knows that she does not consent to it or is reckless as to whether she consents to it.

SEXUAL HARASSMENT IN THE WORKPLACE

Sexual harassment at work is a form of unlawful sex discrimination because the selection of victim is determined by gender. The term encompasses physical, verbal and nonverbal conduct of a sexual nature, for example unwanted touching, repeated brushing up against or attempts to make physical contact with another individual, sexual propositions and innuendo, sexually explicit gestures and the display-ing of offensive material. It is most likely to be perpetrated by men against women and by individuals in high-status jobs, or positions of relative power, against their subordinates. It is unwanted, uninvited, unreciprocated and unwelcome to the recipient who is often personally threatened and intimidated by the behaviour (Mezey and Rubenstein, 1992). To be defined as harassment, the behaviour must be sufficiently serious or persistent to be damaging to the victim's working conditions (Rubenstein, 1989).

Surveys of female employees from several organizations outside the NHS reveal a substantial number of women who report these experiences (US Merit Systems Protection Board, 1988; McCormack, 1985; Mackinnon, 1979; Rubenstein, 1989). Similarly, surveys of health workers confirm widespread accounts of interactions that are considered at best inappropriate and insensitive, at worst abusive and destructive (Garrett and Thomas-Peter, 1992; Glaser and Thorpe, 1986; Baldwin *et al.*, 1991; Wolf *et al.*, 1991; Garvin and Sledge, 1992).

Very few victims of harassment manage to take effective measures to prevent or discourage such behaviour (Gutek, 1985). It is consistently reported that disclosure of harassment often exacerbates the situation and penalizes the victim more than the perpetrator (Tangri *et al.*, 1982). Recent highly publicized cases in the USA and the UK brought by Anita Hill (*The Guardian*, 1991) and Alanah Houston (*The Guardian*, 1992) alleging sexual harassment by colleagues resulted in the public vilification of the victim as well as financial ruin for the women concerned and have done very little to encourage other victims to report similar incidents.

WHAT IS SEXUAL HARASSMENT?

There is considerable misunderstanding about what exactly is meant by sexual harassment. The term is itself often implied to mean over-enthusiastic flirtation or harmless admiration, which is only interpreted as harassment by women who 'cannot take a joke, who are overly sensitive or unreasonably prudish'. There is a tendency to trivialize certain behaviours which, outside the workplace, would constitute criminal assaults and are experienced by the victim as intimidating and humiliating. The perception of a set of interactions as harassment will depend on the interaction between personal variables (e.g. demographic characteristics, personal attitudes, education, past experiences, expectations and attributions) and situational variables (Terpstra and Baker, 1991).

In a recent national opinion poll carried out in the UK, the attitudes and definition of sexual harassment were examined in over 1000 male and female respondents. Both men and women were found to be broadly in agreement with the definition and extent of sexually harassing behaviour. The group tending to criticize the victim most were female respondents over the age of 55 years: this group was most likely to endorse the statement 'most women who complain about sexual harassment have only themselves to blame because of the way they dress and behave' (*The Independent*, 1991). There was otherwise no gender difference in whether particular behaviours constituted harassment or would be acceptable in the workplace. This finding makes it difficult to sustain the argument that men who harass are simply unaware of the unacceptable and inappropriate nature of their behaviour. Other surveys in the USA have suggested that women operate a lower threshold when defining behaviour as harassment, although age may not have been controlled for (Fitzgerald and Ormerod, 1991; Collins and Blodgett, 1981; Kenig and Ryan, 1986).

Clearly there are gradations of harassing behaviours from the subtle innuendo, sexual put-down and teasing comments, to actual and attempted sexual contact, sexual coercion and bribery. If the harassment is perpetrated by a supervisor or boss and involves clear intimidation or coercive sex, there is general consensus about defining the behaviour as harassment. However, very often the behaviour masquerades as affection or friendliness, which the perpetrator uses to justify and neutralize his intentions. More pernicious is the use of powers to employ, promote or fire employees to persuade the employee to have sex and to ensure their continuing loyalty and silence over the matter (MacKinnon, 1979; Mezey and Rubenstein, 1992). Arguably all situations of harassment represent an abuse of an unequal power dynamic. The situations vary in terms of degree rather than implying different motivations or consequences for the victim.

EXPLANATIONS OF SEXUAL HARASSMENT

Tangri and colleagues (1982) have proposed three explanatory models of sexual harassment at work:

1. The natural/biological model attributes sexual harassment to a relatively greater sexual drive in men than women;
2. The organizational model proposes that sexual harassment occurs where the climate of the workplace is one which encourages power/status differentials between male and female workers; and
3. The sociocultural model considers harassment in the workplace as a microcosm of a Western patriarchy where the powerless are exploited and dominated by the relatively powerful members of that society.

It is likely that negative, objectifying and denigrating attitudes to women do not simply arise *de novo* in the workplace. Images of women in traditional roles, as passive, self-effacing and essentially subservient to the men they live and work with will create an expectation of such altruistic and nurturing behaviours in the workplace. These behaviours may be entirely incompatible and aversive to career promotion, creating what has been called the sex-role spillover (Gutek, 1985).

The role of sexuality and sexual attraction in sexual harassment has tended to be underplayed. However, it is likely that a certain amount of harassment starts on the premise of assuming some mutual sexual attraction. Some advances may be a clumsy or insensitive attempt to make some kind of intimate contact, others are opportunistic. The additional presence of alcohol may make certain generally prohibited behaviours between colleagues permissible and serve as a rationale for that individual's apparent loss of control. The relationship between the various models of understanding sexual harassment is likely to be interactive rather than exclusive, different factors having a different impact depending on the individual and specific situation (Gutek and Morasch, 1982; Brewer, 1982).

The dynamics of sexual harassment in the workplace and the sexual exploitation of patients by their carers has parallels with sexual abuse within the family. Both represent an abuse of power and trust and are attributable more to feelings of inadequacy and hostility in the perpetrator than to sexual frustration or unfettered ardour (Pryor, 1987). The end result of sexual harassment is to disadvantage all women, to reinforce the glass ceiling against women's promotion and achievement in the workplace, to encourage lowered expectations and aspirations both for the victim and for the female workforce as a whole. The experience of sexual harassment, even the threat alone may become a means of social control within the workplace by which the male employees' position of economic privilege and status is maintained at the expense of the women's. This dynamic is reminiscent of Susan Brownmiller's description of rape as 'a conscious form of intimidation by which all men keep all women in a state of fear' (Brownmiller, 1976).

EFFECTS OF SEXUAL HARASSMENT

While most women state that they would respond to harassment by confronting the harasser (Terpstra and Baker, 1989), in reality most women either ignore the behaviour or do nothing about it (US Merit Systems Protection Board, 1988). Women are more likely to employ multiple responses to sexual harassment, particularly avoiding behaviours (Benson and Thomson, 1982), while men's reactions are more limited and stereotyped, tending to prefer some kind of physical response (Terpstra and Baker, 1991). Very few individuals take out any formal grievance procedure through their management structure (Gutek, 1985).

While several victims report essentially neutral reactions to the behaviour at the time, there is some evidence that their perceptions become increasingly negative on subsequent appraisal (Glaser and Thorpe, 1986).

Sexual harassment has adverse consequences for the victim's psychological, emotional and physical well-being (Salisbury *et al.*, 1986) The effects parallel the responses of victims of crime; however, the main impacts are on economic and career development with private relationships and physical well-being coming second for victims of harassment at work. The reverse relationship is described for victims of crime (Salisbury *et al.*, 1986). The victim may initially be aware of feelings of tension and general anxiety, a sense of apprehension, certain vague stress-related symptoms, insomnia, increased muscle tension with headaches, physical pains, irritability and poor concentration (Loy and Stewart, 1984; Crull, 1982; Mezey and Rubenstein, 1992; Salisbury *et al.*, 1986). She finds herself dreading coming into work, she finds excuses to avoid work, she experiences impaired concentration, has difficulty in keeping her mind on her work (Crull, 1982; Gutek, 1985). She becomes preoccupied with the possibility of encountering the harasser and in thinking of ways of avoiding being alone with him. The victim may feel ashamed, guilty and contaminated (Gutek, 1985) and may experience a loss of sexual drive and enjoyment (Mezey and Rubenstein, 1992). The working environment is experienced as hostile, unwelcoming, threatening and unsafe.

Continuing harassment may impair the victim's ability to trust, which interferes wth her relationships with others, undermines her confidence and self-esteem and makes her perceive herself as vulnerable and defenceless. If the situation continues, in other words, if the source of stress is not removed, with continuing harassment or the anticipation of unavoidable contact with the harasser, this may lead to mental illness developing including depression, increasing generalized and phobic anxiety, absenteeism from work and post-traumatic stress reactions (Mezey and Rubenstein, 1992). The long-term prospects for the victim of harassment are not good with high rates of job losses, transfers, demotions, lowered wages and poor job references all being reported (Crull, 1982; Gutek, 1985; Terpstra and Cook, 1985; Terpstra and Baker, 1991). There are no similar studies documenting the long-term psychological effects or employment and promotion prospects for the perpetrators, but one suspects there would be few adverse repercussions noted.

The victims of harassment are often less valued by the organization and arguably their services are expendable in contrast to the highly skilled, often highly paid perpetrator. It is therefore not surprising perhaps that companies and organizations often fail to take effective action against individuals accused of harassment and attempt to solve the problem by ridding themselves of the complainant. Having a harasser as an employee has, however, considerable financial consequences for any organization since money is lost: (i) through employees taking additional sick leave; (ii) by replacing those employees during sickness;

(iii) through the retraining and replacing of employees who leave; and (iv) money is also lost through decreased efficiency by the victim should she choose to remain or be unable to leave (US Merit Systems Protection Board, 1988).

The harasser is unlikely to stop his activities simply because the victim leaves: as with sex offenders the tendency to harass and humiliate is related to individual characteristics of the perpetrator (e.g. insecurity, inadequacy, hostility towards and fear of women) rather than to the sexual desirability of the potential victim (Pryor, 1987). Women in the workplace will be targeted if they are perceived as particularly vulnerable and safe in terms of their relative powerlessness and lack of effective voice within the organization, in other words if the perpetrator anticipates that there will be no adverse repercussions for himself.

The question 'why doesn't the victim of sexual harassment simply leave?' is one that is similarly asked of victims of domestic violence and is related to the victim's sense of helplessness and hopelessness, pervasive undermining of the victim's confidence and self-esteem, the failure of the system to heed and respond effectively to repeated cries for help and uncertainty about being able to survive financially in the outside world without the assurance of continuing employment.

SEXUAL VICTIMIZATION OF PATIENTS
BY THEIR CARERS

Sexual relationships between health professionals and their clients are both unethical and potentially damaging to the victim (Fahy and Fisher, 1992; Lazarus, 1992). The activity takes place in a climate of secrecy and shame and represents a violation of trust and professional boundaries.

The sexual abuse of patients by their carers is widely documented, but rarely discussed openly. US surveys suggest that between 5% and 13% of psychiatrists and psychologists acknowledge erotic behaviour with their patients (Holroyd and Brodsky, 1977; Bouhoutsos, 1985; Bouhoutsos *et al.*, 1983; Gartrell *et al.*, 1986, 1989; Herman *et al.*, 1987; Pope and Bouhoutsos, 1986). Obstetricians and nonpsychiatric physicians appear to be particularly prone to engage in sexual relations with their patients (Kardener *et al.*, 1973; Perr, 1989) while psychoanalysts are most unanimous in their condemnation of intimacy with patients as a form of boundary violation (Conte *et al.*, 1989).

Recent, highly publicized cases of the systematic abuse of children in residential homes by their carers have highlighted the need for proper selection and monitoring of individuals who choose to work with particularly vulnerable groups of clients such as children, the mentally and physically disabled and the socially disadvantaged.

As with other forms of sexual abuse, high rates of nondisclosure by the victim are documented and professionals are very reluctant to 'blow the whistle' on their colleagues. In one study, only 8% of therapists who were aware of colleagues' sexual misconduct reported the case to the authorities (Gartrell *et al.*, 1987). Of all complaints made by patients against doctors in the USA, only an estimated 4% were for reasons of sexual impropriety (Pope, 1988). In Britain, the General Medical Council lists annually the figures of complaints made against practitioners, the reasons for these complaints and the outcome of any internal disciplinary procedure. There are similar guidelines defining inappropriate professional conduct for psychologists (DCP, 1990). Both indecency cases and cases involving a personal relationship of an emotional or sexual nature with a patient are grounds for charges of serious professional misconduct. During 1990, the Professional Conduct Committee in the UK heard nine cases of alleged indecency or sexual misconduct towards patients (GMC, 1990). In seven cases the allegations were proven; in two they were not.

Concern about protecting the rights and privacy of the innocent defendant have led to a debate on whether cases of alleged sexual misconduct should be heard in private as opposed to the public forum that operates at the present time. There are no current plans to change procedures and it remains the case that, although these complaints represent a minority of all complaints received, the Council retains the view that:

> ... good medical practice is founded on the maintenance of trust between doctors and patients and it is therefore a most serious matter for a doctor to breach that trust by taking sexual advantage of a patient whom he or she knows to be particularly vulnerable for medical, psychological or social reasons.
>
> (*GMC, 1991*)

In spite of the clear position taken by the GMC, there is little in the training of health professionals that prepares them for the possibility of therapist–patient sexual attraction, let alone the likelihood of sexual intimacy between therapist and patient and there is a clear need for ethical guidelines in relation to this possibility (Folman, 1991). There is a lack of professional debate on whether sexual contact between therapist and patient should be prohibited for all time or simply during the course of professional contact, whether a sexual relationship with a patient can be ethical after termination of treatment and if so, how much time would have to lapse after treatment before it can be said to have ended (Appelbaum and Jorgensen, 1991).

Sexual contact between patients or clients and those entrusted with their care is both unethical and potentially damaging to the victim (Smith and Bisbing, 1987; Fahy and Fisher, 1992; Lazarus, 1992). When an individual consults a health professional, that professional is placed in a position of trust and power relative to the powerlessness and dependency of the patient. Therapeutic interactions are characterized by a recreation and replication of the original parent–child relationship through the emergence of the powerful transferential and countertransferential feelings between the patient and their therapist (Barnhouse, 1978). An ensuing sexual relationship is, at least symbolically, an incestuous one (Bouhoutsos *et al.*, 1983; Pope and Bouhoutsos, 1986). Certain patient populations (e.g. psychiatric patients) represent a particularly disadvantaged group who are even less capable of seeking help and resisting approaches than others and may thus find themselves particularly vulnerable to abuse and exploitation (Gath, 1989).

As in other forms of sexual violence, clinicians who engage in improper behaviour or sexual relationships with their patients are overwhelmingly male, while most victims are female (Perry, 1976; Gartrell *et al.*, 1986). Several female practitioners are reported to engage in nonsexual comfort touching (Perry, 1976), although in practice it may be difficult for the recipients to distinguish erotic from nonerotic contact. Equally, given the fact that the majority of studies of patient sexual abuse are American, there is likely to be a cultural component to defining any physical contact between patient and doctor as abusive. Nonsexual physical contact between therapist and patient may be more acceptable in the USA, for example, than in corresponding clinics and practices in the UK. Although sexual attraction may underlie the behaviour of some abusive therapists, motivations of power and control, anger and aggression appear to be more fundamental needs than the release of sexual desire (Sonne and Pope, 1991). Other explanations for the behaviour include feelings of inadequacy in the therapist, the presence of a mid-life crisis, a need to be loved, depression or alternatively grandiosity, which leads to a feeling of entitlement (Dahlberg, 1970; Kardener, 1974; Folman, 1991). The sexual contact represents one example of an erosion of professional boundaries in an individual who constantly and repeatedly disregards and violates these boundaries in all areas of his practice (Pope and Bouhoutsos, 1986; Kardener *et al.*, 1976; Folman, 1991).

While most physicians believe that sexual contact with a patient is unethical (Herman *et al.*, 1987; Perry, 1976), those who engage in sexual activity tend to justify or rationalize their behaviour (Kardener *et al.*, 1973; Herman *et al.*, 1987; Gartrell *et al.*, 1987; Pope and Bajt, 1988). However, several surveys demonstrate glaring discrepancies between physicians' ethical beliefs and their actual behaviours (Folman, 1991). Psychiatrists who acknowledge sexual contact with patients are significantly more tolerant of such behaviour and more likely to minimize the effects on the victim than nonabusive therapists

(Herman *et al.*, 1987; Pope, 1990). The tendency to justify behaviour that is unequivocally condemned by professional peers has parallels in the excuses used by child molesters to deny their own responsibility and achieve emotional congruence, which allows them to continue abusing children (Finkelhor, 1986; Mezey *et al.*, 1992). For example, sexual contact with a patient is not harmful if it reflects genuine feelings on the part of the therapist.

In a study of 1423 psychiatrists, 84 (6.4%) acknowledged having sexual contact with their patients; the largest number of patients involved with one offender was 12 (Gartrell *et al.*, 1989). Of the offenders, 73% claimed the sexual contact was an expression of love or pleasure, 19% claimed contact would enhance the patient's self-esteem. Other justifications included loss of control, judgement lapse, impulsivity and personal needs. Of the offenders, 65% stated they were in love with the patients, whereas 92% believed that the patients were in love with them. Several offenders (1.6%) reported sexual experiences with their own therapists, female psychiatrists being more likely to have experienced this. While a range of behaviours have been documented, from sexual remarks, to kissing and fondling, sexual intercourse was engaged in by 11% of male physicians in one study of over 400 male physicians but by none of the female physicians (Perry, 1976).

Although most offenders recognize that sexual contact is a means of self-gratification, they are willing to disregard or claim to be unaware of clinical and ethical prohibitions (Bouhoutsos *et al.*, 1983; Gartrell *et al.*, 1987). Erotic practitioners appear able to persuade themselves that their patients' compliance represents genuine willingness and attraction to them (Kardener *et al.*, 1976). This mutuality of sexual attraction is not borne out by testimonies of patients who are abused within a therapeutic context (Sonne and Pope, 1991; Burgess, 1981; Bouhoutsos *et al.*, 1983; Feldman-Summers and Jones, 1984) or by the accounts of abused psychiatrists (Gartrell *et al.*, 1987).

Patients who have been victims of prior sexual abuse or assault appear to be particularly vulnerable to a repetition of this abuse within the therapeutic relationship, which they may originally have entered in order to receive help. Adult survivors of childhood sexual abuse characteristically behave in what is seen as a provocative, flirtatious way in therapy, particularly when the therapist is male (Briere, 1989). Such behaviours represent both a testing out of boundaries with the therapist and a sexualization of nonerotic interactions, which previous experience will have taught as the only effective and legitimate form of interaction with men. It is the responsibility of the therapist not to misinterpret the transference phenomena and re-enact the former abusive relationship within therapy or to personalize the patient's overtures as a manifestation of personal attraction. It is doubtful whether patients are able to give informed consent to sex within the context of a therapeutic relationship; any apparent consent in the context of a doctor–patient relationship is rendered invalid.

The result of the therapists' sexual acting out is that the patient becomes therapeutically orphaned. The caretaker sacrifices the needs or wishes of the patient for his own gratification (Kardener, 1974). Such acting out is additionally likely to lead to impaired decision-making abilities by the patient and pave the way for other abuses such as coercion and fraud (Appelbaum and Jorgensen, 1991).

The psychological and emotional impact on the victim, as well as the extent of the phenomenon, has lead to the description of a patient–therapist sex syndrome in the US literature (Pope, 1988; Pope and Bouhoutsos, 1986), which has parallels with 'rape trauma syndrome' (Burgess and Holmstrom, 1974) and 'battered woman syndrome' (Walker, 1979). Features of 'patient–therapist sex syndrome' include ambivalence, guilt, sexual confusion, impaired ability to trust, identity confusion, emotional lability, anger, suicidal ideation and cognitive dysfunction (Pope, 1988; Pope and Bouhoutsos, 1986). Feldman-Summers and Jones (1984) found that women who had been sexually involved with their therapist were more mistrustful of men and therapists and showed higher levels of anxiety and psychosomatic symptoms than women who had no such experience. The effects of therapists' sexual acting out are likely to be more severe given that the victims already represent a help-seeking population who are likely to have higher rates of pre-existing psychological and social dysfunction.

CONCLUSION

There is clearly a need to recognize the rights of all individuals to seek help from health professionals without fear of abuse, exploitation or violence. There is a need for professionals to recognize that, while sexual attraction may appear to exist between them and their clients, the responsibility for any sexual acting out lies with the professional and their duty of care towards their client. Training bodies for health professionals have a responsibility to discourage sexual harassment and unethical intimacy by raising awareness of the issue (Garrett and Thomas-Peter, 1992) and there have been calls for the criminalization of such behaviours (Strasburger *et al.*, 1991). The victims of such sexual misconduct need understanding, support and the assurance that questions will be asked and organizational policies implemented to prevent such incidents happening again.

REFERENCES

Appelbaum, P.S. and Jorgensen, L. (1991) Psychotherapist–patient sexual contact after termination of treatment. An analysis and a proposal. *American Journal of Psychologists*, **148**(11), 1466–83.

Baldwin, D.C., Daugherty, S.R., and Eckenfels, E.J. (1991) Student perceptions of mistreatment and harassment during medical school. A survey of 10 united schools. *Western Journal of Medicine*, **155**(2), 140–45.

Barnhouse, R.T. (1978) Sex between patient and therapist. *Journal of American Academy of Psychoanalysis*, **6**, 533–44.

Benson, D.J. and Thomson, G.E. (1982) Sexual harassment on a university campus: The confluence of authority relations, sexual interest and gender stratification. *Social Problems*, **29**, 236–51.

Bouhoutsos, J. (1985) Therapist–client sexual involvement: A challenge for mental health professionals and educators. *American Journal of Orthopsychiatry*, **55**, 177–82.

Bouhoutsos, J., Holroyd, J., Lerman, H. *et al.* (1983) Sexual intimacy between psychotherapists and patients. *Professional Psychology*, **14**, 185–96.

Brewer, M.B. (1982) Further beyond nine to five: An integration and future directions. *Journal of Social Issues*, **38**, 149–58.

Briere, J. (1989) *Therapy for Adults Molested as Children*, Springer, New York.

Brownmiller, S. (1976) *Against Our Will. Men, Women and Rape*, Penguin, London.

Burgess, A.W. (1981) Physician sexual misconduct and patient responses. *American Journal of Psychiatry*, **138**(10), 1335–42.

Burgess, A.W. and Holmstrom, L. (1974) Rape trauma syndrome. *American Journal of Psychiatry*, **137**, 981–88.

Collins, E.G.C. and Blodgett, T.B. (1981) Sexual harassment – some see it, some won't. *Harvard Business Review*, **59**, 76–95.

Conte, H., Plutchik, R., Picard, S. *et al.* (1989) Ethics in the practice of psychotherapy. *American Journal of Psychotherapy*, **43**, 32–42.

Crull, P. (1982) Stress effects of sexual harassment on the job: Implications for counselling. *American Journal of Orthopsychiatry*, **52**, 539–44.

Dahlberg, C. (1970) Sexual contact between patient and therapist. *Contemporary Psycho Analysis*, **6**, 107–24.

DCP (1990) *Guidelines for the Professional Practice of Clinical Psychology*, The British Psychological Society, Leicester.

Fahy, T. and Fisher, S. (1992) Sexual contact between doctors and patients – almost always harmful. *British Medical Journal*, **304**, 1519–20.

Feldman-Summers, S. and Jones, G. (1984) Psychological impact of sexual contact between therapists or other health care professionals and their clients. *Journal of Consulting and Clinical Psychology*, **52**, 1054–61.

Finkelhor, D. (1986) *A Sourcebook on Child Sexual Abuse*, Sage, Beverly Hills.

Fitzgerald, L.F. and Ormerod, A.J. (1991) Perceptions of sexual harassment. The influence of gender and academic context. *Psychology of Women Quarterly*, **15**, 281–94.

Folman, R.Z. (1991) Therapist–patient sex: Attraction and boundary problems. *Psychotherapy*, **28**(1), 168–73.

Garrett, T., and Thomas-Peter, B. (1992) Sexual harassment. *Psychologist*, July, 19–21.

Gartrell, M., Herman, J., Olarte, S. *et al.* (1986) Psychiatrist–patient sexual contact: results of a national survey. I: Prevalence. *American Journal of Psychiatry*, **143**(9) 1126–1131.

Gartrell, M., Herman, J., Olarte, S., *et al.* (1987) Reporting practises of psychiatrists who knew of sexual misconduct by colleagues. *American Journal of Ortho Psychiatry*, **57**(2), 287–95.

Gartrell, M., Herman, J., Olarte, S. *et al.* (1989) Prevalence of psychiatrist–patient sexual contact, in *Sexual Exploitation in Professional Relationships*, (ed. G.O. Gabbard), APP, Washington DC.

Garvin, C. and Sledge, S.H. (1992) Sexual harassment within dental offices in Washington State. *Journal of Dental Hygiene*, **66**(4), 178–84.

Gath, A. (1989) Statement on abuse and harassment within psychiatric hospitals. *Psychiatric Bulletin*, **13**, 460.

Glaser, R.D. and Thorpe, J.S. (1986) Unethical intimacy: A survey of sexual contact and advances between psychology educators and female graduate students. *American Psychologist*, **41**(1), 43–51.

GMC (1990) *Annual Report 1990*, General Medical Council, London.

GMC (1991) *Annual report 1991*, General Medical Council, London.

Guardian, The, (1991) 15 October, *Fallacy of a Flirters Charter*.

Guardian, The, (1992) 13 May, *Life Amongst the Ruins Left by Law*.

Gutek, B. (1985) *Sex and the Workplace*, Jossey-Bass, San Francisco.

Gutek, B.A. and Morasch, B. (1982) Sex ratios, sex role spillover and sexual harassment at work. *Journal of Social Issues*, **38**(4), 55–74.

Herman, J.L., Gartrell, M., Olarte, S. *et al.* (1987) Psychiatrist–patient sexual contact: results of a national survey. II: Psychiatrists' attitudes. *American Journal of Psychiatry*, **144**(2), 164–69.

Holroyd, J.C. and Brodsky, A.M. (1977) Psychologists attitudes and practises regarding erotic and nonerotic physical contact with patients. *American Journal of Psychologists*, **32**, 843–49.

Independent, The, (1991) 20 October, *Sexes Agree on Harassed Women*.

Kardener, S.H. (1974) Sex and the physician patient relationship. *American Journal of Psychologists*, **131**(10), 1134–36.

Kardener, S.H., Fuller, M. and Mensh, I.N. (1973) A survey of physicians' attitudes and practices regarding erotic and nonerotic contact with patients. *American Journal of Psychologists*, **130**, 1077–81.

Kardener, S.H., Fuller, M. and Mensh, I.N. (1976) Characteristics of (erotic) practitioners. *American Journal of Psychologists*, **133**(1), 1324–25.

Kenig, S. and Ryan, J. (1986) Sex difference in levels of tolerance and attribution of blame for sexual harassment on a university campus. *Sex Roles*, **15**, 535–49.

Lazarus, J.A. (1992) Sex with former patients almost always unethical. *American Journal of Psychologists*, **149**(7), 855–57.

Loy, P.H. and Stewart, L.P. (1984) The extent and effects of the sexual harassment of working women. *Sociological Focus*, **17**(1), 31–43.

MacKinnon, C. (1979) *Sexual Harassment of Working Women. A Case of Sex Discrimination*, New Haven, Connecticut.

McCormack, A. (1985) The sexual harassment of students by teachers: The case of students in science. *Sex Roles*, **13**, 21–32.

Mezey, G. and Rubenstein, M. (1992) Medicolegal aspects of sexual harassment. *Journal of Forensic Psychiatry*, **3**(2), 221–33.

Mezey, G., Vizard, E., Hawkes, C. *et al.* (1992) A community treatment programme for convicted child sex offenders: A preliminary report. *Journal of Forensic Psychiatry*, **2**, 11–25.

Perr, I.N. (1989) Medicolegal aspects of professional sexual exploitation, in *Sexual Exploitation in Professional Relationships*, (ed. G.O. Gabbard), APP, Washington DC.

Perry, J.A. (1976) Physicians' erotic and nonerotic physical involvement with patients. *American Journal of Psychologists*, **133**(7), 838–40.

Pope, I. and Bouhoutsos, J. (1986) *Sexual Intimacies Between Patients and Therapists*, Praeger, New York.

Pope, K.F. (1988) How clients are harmed by sexual contact with mental health professionals: The syndrome and its prevalence. *Journal of Counselling and Development*, **67**, 222–26.

Pope, K.F. and Bajt, T.R. (1988) When laws and values conflict, dilemma for psychologists. *American Journal of Psychologists*, **43**, 828–29.

Pope, K.S. (1990) Therapist patient sex as sex abuse: Scientific professional and practical dilemmas in addressing victimization and rehabilitation. *Professional Psychology: Research and Practice*, **21**, 227–39.

Pryor, J.B. (1987) Sexual harassment proclivities in men. *Sex Roles*, **17**, 269–90.

Rubenstein, M. (1989) *Preventing and Remedying Harassment at Work: A Resource Manual*, Industrial Relation Services, London.

Salisbury, J., Ginorio, A., Remick, H. *et al.* (1986) Counselling victims of sexual harassment. *Psychotherapy*, **23**(2), 316–24.

Smith, J. and Bisbing, S. (1987) Sexual exploitation of patients: The civil, criminal and professional consequences. *Trial*, 65–70.

Sonne, J.L. and Pope, K.F. (1991) Treating victims of therapist–patient sexual involvement. *Psychotherapy*, **28**(1), 174–87.

Strasburger, L.H., Jorgenson, L. and Rundles, R. (1991) Criminalization of psychotherapist–patient sex. *American Journal of Psychologists*, **148**, 859–63.

Tangri, S., Burt, R.M. and Johnson, L.B. (1982) Sexual harassment at work: Three explanatory models. *Journal of Social Issues*, **38**, 33–54.

Terpstra, D.E. and Baker, D.D. (1989) The identification and classification of reactions to sexual harassment. *Journal of Organisational Behaviour*, **10**(1), 1–14.

Terpstra, D.E. and Baker, D.D. (1991) Sexual harassment at work: The psychosocial issues, in *Vulnerable Workers: Psychosocial and Legal Issues*, (eds M. Davidson and G. Earnshaw), John Wiley, Chichester.

Terpstra, D.E. and Cook, S.E. (1985) Complainant characteristics and reported behaviours and consequences associated with formal sexual harassment charges. *Personnel Psychology*, **38**(3), 559–74.

US Merit Systems Protection Board (1988) *Sexual Harassment in the Federal Government: Is it a problem?* US Government Printing Office, Washington DC.

Walker, L.E.A. (1979) *The Battered Woman*, Harper and Row, New York.

Wolf, T.M., Randall, H.M., Von Almen, K. *et al.* (1991) Perceived mistreatment and attitude by graduating medical students: A retrospective study. *Medical Education*, **25**(3), 182–90.

PART TWO

Reactions to violence

CHAPTER 6

Reactions to assault

Til Wykes and Richard Whittington

INTRODUCTION

The first few chapters in this book set out the risks of violence in different groups and for different settings. Much attention has been given to the perpetrators of this violence. Their social and demographic characteristics, diagnoses if any and the sorts of triggers for their acts of violence have been investigated in detail. In contrast, little attention has been given to the victims. This chapter will try to redress the balance by concentrating not on questions of who gets involved or why but on the after effects in the highly trained and dedicated group of workers who sometimes have to suffer in silence.

Violence not only involves physical force with the intent to harm but can also include verbal aggression and threats to harm. Nevertheless, from the observer's point of view, the extent of injury is generally conceived in terms of the physical damage to the victim. Undoubtedly the level of injury affects the reactions but when there are no physical signs this does not mean that there are few effects. In fact Conn and Lion (1983) found that 'almost unanimously the victims of assault agreed that the emotional impact of the incident far exceeded the impact of the physical injury'.

VIOLENCE IN THE COMMUNITY

Much of the information about the effects of violence comes from studies on the effects of violent crime. The crimes covered include robbery, wounding, physical assault and homicide. The evidence on victimization (the effects of being a victim) is provided mainly by the British Crime Survey, which tended to focus on less serious offences (Hough and Mayhew, 1985) and an interview study carried out by Shapland *et al.* (1985), which concentrated on more serious offences.

Overall in 26% of wounding cases extra worry, fear or loss of confidence were reported, 11% reported depression, stress or sleep problems and 5% were considerably upset. The most conservative estimates suggest some sort of psychological support is required for about one in four victims of crimes excluding rape (Maguire and Corbett, 1987). These figures are affected by whether the victim knew the offender well. If they did the incidence of being seriously affected went up to 51% (Mawby and Gill, 1987).

Very few crimes of rape or woman battering were included in the above studies but it is recognized that these crimes are bound to have serious psychological sequelae. The rape trauma syndrome (Burgess and Holmstrom, 1974), although it may follow different time courses for different individuals, is widely acknowledged as occurring in most women who have experienced rape. It is a crime that is recognized as having a very toxic effect on psychological well-being when compared with other crimes. This extra toxic effect occurs even when the effects of violence and dangerousness of the crime have been controlled (Kilpatrick *et al.*, 1989).

Physical injuries can be sustained in several ways; this may have a psychological impact. However, it is our view that the cause of injuries, for example by an accident or violent assault, provides a major contribution to their traumatic effects. Some supporting evidence comes from a study in which a series of 122 people with jaw fractures in a casualty department were interviewed about their reactions following the injury. The accident victims differed little from those who were the victims of assault either in their personalities prior to their injury or in their reactions in the first week after it. However, when tested at 3 months, the assault victims showed more depression and anxiety than those who sustained their injuries in an accident (Shepherd *et al.*, 1990).

Breslau and colleagues investigated the lifetime prevalence of severe disorder (post-traumatic stress disorder, PTSD) following traumatic events in a population survey of 1007 young adults in Detroit (Breslau *et al.*, 1991). Their results add weight to the distinction between types of traumatic events (Table 6.1). The lowest rate of PTSD was found in the accident and injury cases and, with the exception of rape, the other categories (which included assault) had approximately the same prevalence. It is interesting to note that 75% of people who had experienced traumatic events (apart from rape) were unaffected by the disorder although they could have suffered from other less disabling conditions. Breslau and colleagues also showed that there were other psychological conditions associated with PTSD such as obsessive-compulsive disorder, major depression, panic and agoraphobia.

All these studies show that the victims of violence show similar effects that are far more intense than might have been predicted from

Table 6.1 Prevalence of PTSD by type of event[a]

Type of traumatic event	Prevalence of PTSD
Physical assault	23%
Seeing someone killed or seriously injured	24%
Hearing the news of sudden death or accident of close relative, friend or spouse	21%
Threat to life	24%
Rape	80%
Sudden injury or serious accident	12%

[a] Source: adapted from Breslau *et al.*, 1991.

a simple examination of the physical injury. Victims often feel helpless, out of control, depressed, ashamed, anxious, frightened and disorganized. They also show behavioural changes such as sleep problems, uncontrollable crying, restlessness, deterioration of personal relationships and an increase in the use of drugs. Some of these symptoms may have resolved within 6 months of the event but, for some victims, the psychological consequences are severe and long-lasting. These effects are best viewed as 'normal' responses to trauma falling into the descriptive category of PTSD. The only factor that is likely to distinguish these victims from those of natural disasters is that the effects are worse when the traumatic events are human-induced and intended by the perpetrator (Janoff-Bulman, 1988).

Other research on the effects of violent crime has tried to identify which factors are most important in developing psychological problems. The presence of physical injury and life threat have both been identified as increasing the risk of developing a serious psychiatric disorder, known as 'crime-related PTSD' (Kilpatrick *et al.*, 1989.

Symptoms may also abate at different rates for different individuals. Studies of the course of symptoms following rape have shown that 94% of victims have severe psychological reactions but 3 months after the event only 47% of victims show the severe psychological reactions and some victims (16.5%) show these effects for some considerable time.

In summary, research on the effects of violence in the community has shown that there are psychological reactions that are worse if the person has been injured via an assault rather than through an accident. These reactions are affected mainly by:

- knowing the perpetrator;
- the extent of the injury;
- whether there was a threat to life; and
- the amount of time lapsed following the event.

VIOLENCE IN THE WORKPLACE

Violence at work is not unknown and it is now recognized as an occupational hazard (Chapter 1). Some of the violence at work has similar epidemiology to violence in the community and is not related to the type of work carried out. In this category is the level of maxillofacial injuries at work, which was recently estimated as 0.37 per 1000 workers. Of these cases, 11% were due to assault and battery. Other violence is related either to the type of work, for example handling money, or the organization of work, for example transport employees working single-handed and at night. In a study of work-related homicide in Canada the highest rates occurred amongst policemen, taxi drivers and petrol-station attendants, in other words those working alone. In half the cases the motive was robbery.

Although it is difficult to translate the overall levels to a British context, it is clear that violence occurs at work. However, there are few research studies on the effects of workplace violence on the victims. Surveys of industries such as public tranport and the banking industry have, however, suggested that there are serious effects (Fisher and Jacoby, 1992; Banking and Finance Union, 1993). Police officers who had been involved in disasters or who had been the victims of violence during their work have also been found to suffer severe psychological disturbances which have wide-ranging and negative consequences for the officer and the force (Duckworth, 1990).

As well as similarities with violence in the community there are additional factors that will affect the reactions to violence in a work setting. For instance, avoiding the place where the violence occurred may have serious implications for personal finances. These financial considerations may deter the victim from avoidance and therefore contribute to increased levels of anxiety. Conversely any financial difficulties resulting from avoidance may have an additive effect on the levels of stress experienced.

EXPERIENCES OF HEALTH CARE WORKERS

The levels of violence to staff throughout the health care services have become unacceptable. As many of the authors in this book have pointed out, the violence affects every health care occupation from ambulance staff, casualty departments and general practitioners to community nurses and all staff in psychiatric hospitals. The level of severe violence is low but staff still have to cope with the threat of aggression or actual assault every day. The effects on staff are similar to those on other people who experience violence in the context of work but the particular role of the health care professional as a carer must also have an effect on the outcome.

Many health care workers are trained to recognize and to teach people to cope with psychological distress and this therefore makes them a knowledgeable group of workers. However, this knowledge may not help them to cope with the psychological effects of being involved in a violent incident themselves. The reasons for this are two-fold:

1. the ethos of carers is that they should be able to handle powerful emotions and this leads to denial of the effects and inadequate emotional processing; and
2. tolerance of violence in the workplace leads to the assumption that it is all part of the job and that staff should not make a fuss.

Shouksmith and Wallis (1988) suggest that '(psychiatric nurses) may be disproportionately less likely to recognize or more reluctant to admit mild psychiatric symptoms because of their preoccupation with severely disordered patients and the professional image of themselves as psychologically very well balanced'. This quote probably applies to all staff in the health professions. There is evidence that although symptoms may not be recognized by health care workers, when prompted, they report similar symptoms to those reported by the victims of crime.

SPECIFIC SYMPTOMS

Some symptoms experienced by health care professionals are detailed below. In choosing this approach it was hoped to help victims and their colleagues to identify and empathize. Some of these are from published accounts, others are from our own experiences of victims. We have endeavoured not to exploit victims' accounts and they have only been included where it is helpful in acknowledging their effects on work. Not all of these symptoms will be experienced by every individual involved in a violent incident.

Anxiety

The victim may feel physical signs that indicate anxiety such as butterflies in the stomach, pains in the chest, dry mouth, palpitations, profuse sweating, etc. Often these are worse when the victim is talking about the incident, when they are in the vicinity of the place where the assault took place, or with their assailant.

It is often difficult for victims to cope with these feelings as, generally, they will have to return to the place where the incident occurred and often face their assailant. The symptoms may interfere with their ability to concentrate on their work and make them embarrassed in front of colleagues, patients or clients.

> Carole Protheroe had an ashtray thrown in her face by a young client in a police station. Both eyes were blacked, her glasses broken and her tooth chipped. She reports, 'I had to fight considerable feelings of panic when I had further contact with the client, including the prospect of meeting him in town. Even 6 months later I cannot be entirely sure that anxiety has left me – a visit to a police station can bring sweat to my palms.'
>
> *(Protheroe, 1987)*

Fears and phobias

Some people develop specific fears related to the circumstances of the threat. For instance, if the attack took place within a particular building the victim might find it particularly difficult to re-enter that building. Sometimes these fears generalize to other situations so that any tall building is avoided or the victim finds it hard to work with any men. These sorts of phobias may become so severe that the victim fears leaving their own home.

Cognitive effects

Owing to the anxiety experienced, there are often effects on memory and concentration. The interference from intrusive thoughts is also likely to affect concentration but the relative contributions of intrusive thoughts and high arousal to cognitive difficulties are not yet known.

The victim may find it difficult to follow a television programme or read a newspaper and remember its contents. These lapses of attention can interfere with work performance and may reinforce the worker's feelings of incompetence. This is an area about which little is known except that when cognitive symptoms are severe it is more likely that a long-lasting and disabling condition will develop (Wykes, 1993).

Guilt and self-blame

Although the victim may acknowledge the chance factors in an incident, they may feel partly to blame and this then leads to feelings of guilt and ruminations about how the situation could have been prevented. This belief may be perpetuated by the social group. Some health care workers think that victims are more authoritarian, more provocative, incompetent, demanding, inflexible and incapable of detecting signs of violence (Lanza, 1984, 1987; Poster and Ryan, 1989; Rowett, 1986).

This stereotype is useful to groups who are likely to be at risk of violence because it allows them to assume that becoming a victim is under some control and therefore it follows that so long as they do not possess the qualities associated with the stereotype they will be safe. The victim too is likely to have held such a stereotype and so will question their own abilities more keenly following an assault and accept more responsibility for it. Together with colleagues' doubts, there is set up a cycle of victimization that can reinforce feelings of guilt and self-blame.

Not all feelings of self-blame may be counter-productive. The positive worth of behavioural self-blame has been emphasized by Abramson *et al.* (1978) and by Janoff-Bulman (1988). Behaviour can be changed and this belief can provide the victim with a way of preventing attacks in the future. If the victim begins to blame his or her own character, which is unlikely to change, then this produces a pessimistic outlook. It can only lead to a poor view of self-worth and an expectation of assaults in the future.

> I felt self critical, despising myself for not being more skilful, resourceful and brave.
>
> *(Powell, 1983, cited in Brown et al., 1986)*

> After threatening to murder her the man was arrested and put on remand. The social worker victim reported 'I felt worried that if he wasn't in prison, I might be at risk. So I felt a bit guilty in a sense that I wanted him locked up. I think it's against a social worker's nature to want her client locked up. But I felt quite guilty that I wanted it and glad that he probably was going to be'.
>
> *(Bute, 1979)*

Anger and morbid hatred

Although post-traumatic reactions are categorized as part of the anxiety disorders in the Diagnostic and Statistical Manual – DSMIIIr, it is interesting that one of the reactions that commonly occurs is anger, which occasionally develops into morbid hatred. The anger can be directed at colleagues for not preventing the incident or for not intervening appropriately. Perhaps the most distressing for health professionals is the anger directed towards the perpetrator – especially if this is someone with whom they have to continue a caring relationship.

This anger is sometimes so consuming that the victim thinks about the incident nearly all the time and remains in a state of high arousal. Sometimes the victim has violent dreams that may be of the incident or of related themes.

Outbursts of anger that are not directed towards anyone who was involved in the incident can occur. There is often an increase in irritability, which unfortunately is often felt by the family and friends of the victim, who are just the ones who are called upon to provide help and support.

> John is a male nurse who was assaulted by an elderly woman in a residential home when he offered her night medication. He received a black eye and injuries to his neck and back. He did not feel angry towards the client. However, for over a year he was extremely embittered towards his employers. He thought that they should have foreseen the problem and redirected this woman to a more structured psychiatric setting (which eventually happened). He became completely obsessed with trying to get justice from his employers and was unable to think constructively about the incident. Atlthough he was aroused he seemed to get a sense of satisfaction from his brooding.

> 'I realized in retrospect that I had been very angry, although I had ducked the issue of direct anger towards the client. It is very hard for a social worker to acknowledge extremely punitive feelings! Nevertheless I felt generalized anger at being treated as an object, at being hit because of what I represented rather than as a person'

> *(Protheroe, 1987)*

THE RESPONSE CYCLE

Responses to violent incidents seem to follow a phasic course, with each phase taking differing amounts of time depending on several factors in the situation. Not every person will experience every phase or the phase may be so brief that it is hardly noticeable. Also not every person experiences adverse consequences following an incident but it should be stressed that this is unusual. If this occurs it should not lull the individual or their employers into thinking that the event was not serious. The severity and the implications for ways of working must be considered separately from the effects on the victim.

The phases following violence or the threat of violence at work are: (i) impact; (ii) recoil; and (iii) reorganization.

Impact

Initially the response is a physiological one with high levels of arousal. The victim may be responding to external demands, such as keeping control of the situation and it may be some hours before the actual impact of the event is apparent. This initial constellation of reactions includes shock, numbness, confusion, disorientation, heightened feelings of fear, vulnerability, helplessness, dependency and anger. Appetite change, sleep loss and related fatigue are common, as well as phobic avoidance of reminders of the incident.

Recoil

The immediate aftermath and shock over the incident has passed and now victims learn to deal with powerful emotions. The victim's sense of security is shattered and he or she searches for reasons for their involvement. Pre-incident events are often identified as omens and signs because no answer is immediately available to the 'why me?' question. The victim struggles to gain control so that a re-occurrence can be prevented.

There is often a preoccupation with the incident in this phase so that person needs to talk about it all the time. However, on the other end of the continuum, victims also deny both emotions and thoughts related to the event. Although the temporary use of denial is not pathological because there is a need to rest between bouts of processing, it is likely that continued avoidance increases the time spent in the recoil phase.

Reorganization

This is a calmer phase and it can take considerable time for victims to gain control of their emotions. The golden rule in this phase is that it always takes longer than the victim estimates. The incident is never forgotten but it does not haunt the victim's daily life. The individual is now able to discuss the experience and its meaning. Some victims find that they are stronger for having survived the incident and the resulting emotions. They may feel more resilient to stresses and more able to cope with them. Others may, however, retain only a tenuous ability to cope and may experience relapses each time they are exposed to further stress.

The phases described above are very similar for every incident despite the different professional groups involved and the different situations in which the violence was perpetrated. Although the examples were of actual assaults, most of the violence faced by people at work is not so severe and mainly consists of verbal and physical abuse. Any actual assaults usually result in little or no injury (Whittington and Wykes, 1992; BASW, 1988; D'Urso and Hobbs, 1989; also see Chapters 1 to 4 in this book). However, despite the lack of physical severity, these incidents still have effects on the victim, which can range from acute stress reactions to a disorder that is so severe that it seems indistinguishable from post-traumatic stress disorder (Whittington and Wykes, 1989; Lanza, 1983).

RESEARCH ON HEALTH CARE WORKERS

One of the first studies to look specifically at the effects of violence on health professionals was carried out by Lanza (1983) on 40 nurses who had been involved in an assault. The data were retrospective questionnaires filled out up to 1 year following the assault and therefore they depend on memories of symptoms. Interestingly, half the sample reported minimal reactions to the assault, which Lanza attributes to denial. In fact she went further and suggested that:

> some staff felt that they would be overwhelmed if they allowed themselves to admit to their feelings. Some stated that if they allowed themselves to experience feelings about the likelihood of assault they would not be able to function. Others felt that they had no right to react since being assaulted was part of the job.
> *(Lanza, 1983)*

Some support for the clouding of symptoms through denial by the victim was found by Whittington and Wykes (1989, 1992). In their prospective study, the hospital staff victims often reported that they did not think they had been affected when their symptomatic profiles showed otherwise.

Rowett (1986) surveyed 560 social services staff and found that 60 had been assaulted in the last 3 years. Rowett asked the social workers to report their primary emotions at the time of the assault. The sort of responses were shock, anger, fear, surprise and panic. Only three social workers reported that they were unmoved by the violence. One tenth (10%) reported that it had a permanent effect on their confidence in addition to 18% who said that it had a temporary effect.

Two prospective studies, one in the USA and one in the UK, have now been published which overcome the problems of memory for the symptoms at the time of the assault. These were both carried out in hospitals with the focus on nursing staff. In the UK study, the first 3 weeks following an assault were investigated. Subjects experienced fatigue and irritability as their main problems initially as well as headaches, a desire to smoke and drink more alcohol and more general anxiety. However, they began to awake at night and experience nightmares by the final interview. Most people had experienced less anxiety and 'strain' by 3 weeks following the assault but a few people reported higher levels at the end of the survey than they had initially, which may indicate a short-term delayed effect (Whittington and Wykes, 1989, 1992). Ryan and Poster (1989) in the USA, using similar methodology, were able to follow their victims for a greater length of time. They divided victims into: (i) nonresponders; and (ii) responders on the Assault Response Questionnaire. They followed up the victims for 1 year and showed that the categories of responses most often reported were emotional and biophysiological. The most common emotional response was anger, which was experienced by about half the sample in the week following the assault. The number of responders reduced over time from 67% at week 1 to only 22% at 1 year follow-up. There is also some evidence of a delay in responding. The report does not provide data on the numbers of responders overall but it is clear that at least two-thirds of victims, and probably more, experienced severe effects and that a fifth were still experiencing severe effects at 1 year.

A further study by Flannery and colleagues (Flannery *et al.*, 1991) primarily on the effectiveness of intervention for the effects of violence reported that one of the victims left work in the first 90 days of the programme as a direct result of experiencing an assault. Their treated victims reported fright, anger and apprehension. Sleep disturbance, intrusive memories and hypervigilance were also reported. They also described several occasions during counselling when the victims reported thinking about previous painful incidents in their lives.

These studies, mainly on nurses, have found a similar prevalence of problems. Lanza (1983) found that 30% of her sample identified 22 responses in the short term, Ryan and Poster (1989) found that between 20% and 50% of their sample identified 21 similar responses

Table 6.2 Symptoms identified by research studies on health care workers in the 10 days following assault

Symptom	Research studies identifying this symptom[a]
Shock, disbelief	1,2,4
Anger, irritability	1,2,4,5
Anxiety	1,2,3,5
Helplessness	1,2
Sadness, depression	1,2,3,5
Feeling sorry for the aggressor	1,2
Feeling responsible for the assault	1,2
Hyperalertness	1,2,5
Intrusive thoughts	3,5
Ruminations	3,5
Desire for alcohol, food or drugs	3
Headaches	3
Soreness	1,2
Fatigue	3
Muscle tenseness	3

[a]Data from: 1 = Lanza (1983, 1984), 2 = Poster and Ryan (1989), 3 = Whittington and Wykes (1989, 1992), 4 = Rowett (1986), 5 = Wykes (1993).

and Whittington and Wykes (1992) showed that 25 items were identified in the 3 weeks covering their study. A comparison of the sorts of symptoms that are identified by studies on the effects of violence on health care workers is given in Table 6.2.

PSYCHOLOGICAL REACTIONS – THEORIES ABOUT THE DEVELOPMENT OF PSYCHOPATHOLOGY

Objective stimulus factors

These theories attribute reactions directly to the characteristics of a stimulus, in other words, there is a causal relationship between 'extreme' stimuli and responses. The first of these responses to be described in detail is the **stress response syndrome** (Horowitz, 1986). He proposes that there is a generalized response to traumatic events that is not specific to particular stimuli. The syndrome is characterized by alternating states of denial and intrusion. The signs and symptoms of each of these initial phases are as follows:

1. Denial phase:
    (a) Perception/Attention
       – Daze
       – Selective inattention
       – Inability to appreciate significance of stimuli
       – Amnesia (complete or partial);
    (b) Ideational Processing
       – Disavowal of meanings of stimuli
       – Inflexibility of the organization of thought
       – Fantasies to counteract reality;
    (c) Emotional Reactions
       – Numbness;
    (d) Somatic Reactions
       – Tension-inhibition type symptoms;
    (e) Actions
       – Frantic overactivity to withdrawal;
2. Intrusive phase:
    (a) Perception/Attention
       – Hypervigilance, startle reactions
       – Sleep and dream disturbances;
    (b) Consciousness
       – Intrusive-repetitive thoughts and behaviours (e.g. illusions, pseudo-hallucinations, nightmares, ruminations, repetitions);

(c) Ideational Processing
- Over-generalization
- Inability to concentrate on other topics (preoccupation)
- Confusion and disorganization;

(d) Emotional Reactions
- Emotional attacks or 'pangs';

(e) Somatic Reactions
- Symptomatic sequelae of chronic flight and fight readiness (or of exhaustion);

(f) Actions
- Search for lost persons and situations, compulsive repetitions.

Subsequent work on the longer term symptoms of veterans of the Vietnam war has led to the recognition of a further disabling consequence of traumatic events which has been labelled post-traumatic stress disorder (PTSD) (American Psychiatric Association, 1989). The various criteria for a diagnosis of PTSD are shown in the list following and include symptoms of: (i) high arousal (irritability, difficulty falling asleep); (ii) avoidance (avoiding situations that compel recall of the event) and (iii) re-experiencing (flashbacks). The diagnostic criteria in DSMIIIr for post-traumatic stress disorder (American Psychiatric Association, 1989) are:

1. The person has experienced an event that is outside the range of usual human experience and that would be markedly distressing to almost anyone, e.g. serious threat to one's life or physical integrity;

2. The traumatic event is persistently re-experienced in at least one of the following ways:
   (a) Recurrent and intrusive distressing recollections of the event
   (b) Recurrent distressing dreams of the event
   (c) Sudden acting or feeling as if the traumatic event were recurring (includes a sense of reliving the experience, illusions, hallucinations and dissociation (flashback) episodes, even those that occur upon awakening or when intoxicated)
   (d) Intensive psychological distress at exposure to the events that symbolize or resemble an aspect of the traumatic event, including anniversaries of the trauma;

3. Persistent avoidance of stimuli associated with the trauma or numbing of general responsiveness (not present before the trauma), as indicated by at least three of the following:
   (a) Efforts to avoid thoughts or feelings associated with the trauma
   (b) Efforts to avoid activities or situations that arouse recollections of the trauma

    (c) Inability to recall an important part of the trauma (psychogenic amnesia)

    (d) Markedly diminished interest in significant activities

    (e) Feeling of detachment or estrangement from others

    (f) Restricted range of affect, e.g. unable to have loving feelings

    (g) Sense of foreshortened future, e.g. does not expect to have a career, marriage or children, or a long life;

4. Persistent symptoms of increased arousal (not present before the trauma), as indicated by at least two of the following:

    (a) Difficulty falling or staying asleep

    (b) Irritability or outbursts of anger

    (c) Difficulty concentrating

    (d) Hypervigilance

    (e) Exaggerated startle response

    (f) Physiological reactivity upon exposure to events that symbolize or resemble an aspect of the traumatic event (e.g. a woman who was raped in a lift breaks out into a sweat when entering a lift);

5. Duration of disturbance of symptoms 2–4 of at least 1 month.

These symptoms may be experienced singly and in combination and may not reach the severity or chronicity thresholds required for a diagnosis of PTSD. When symptoms have lasted for more than 1 month and less than 6 months the disorder is described as acute, whereas if there are symptoms past this 6 month threshold then the condition is termed chronic.

Owing to the generality of the responses and the lack of stimulus specificity when the events are severe, the psychological reactions to traumatic events have been described as 'normal reactions to abnormal events'. Not all the symptoms listed are experienced, rather the theory suggests that some symptoms from each section will be experienced at varying times in the initial phases of the disorder.

One further parallel theory is of relevance here, the theory of emotional processing proposed by Rachman (1980). He tried to integrate a disparate set of clinical and experimental observations on the responses to fear-inducing events. He defined emotional processing as a means whereby emotional disturbances are absorbed and decline to the extent that other experiences and behaviour can continue without disruption. There are no clear guidelines on detecting successful emotional processing, only ones for detecting unsuccessful processing. Some of these indices are: (i) pressure of talk; (ii) hallucinations (e.g. after bereavement); (iii) preoccupations; (iv) restlessness; (v) irritability; and (vi) inappropriate expression of emotions (e.g. crying). Many of these signs overlap with Horowitz's stress response syndrome and the diagnostic criteria for PTSD but they were devised in response to less traumatic stimuli. The stressor criterion for PTSD (that the event should be **life-threatening** and outside the range of normal experience) has been questioned by Breslau and Davis (1987). Some supporting evidence comes from a study by Solomon and Canino (1989). They compared the reactions to specific disasters and common stressful events (e.g. moving, money problems, illness, etc.) and found that the reactions to common events were closely related to PTSD symptoms. However, their disaster victims showed significantly higher levels of generalized anxiety than nondisaster victims, even after controlling for other negative life events. This study suggests two conclusions that are relevant to the experience of violence at work. The first is to call into question the emphasis on PTSD as the sole or even major outcome of exposure to traumatic events. This would mean that it would be possible to relate many different disabling psychological reactions **causatively** to the trauma. This is particularly important for the assessment of compensation. The second conclusion is that common events that do not fall outside the range of experience could produce very disabling symptomatology. Certainly it has been our experience that minor assaults at work appear to have long-lasting effects, resulting in phobias, depression and anxiety disorders as well as PTSD.

Rachman (1980) tried to define stimulus characteristics that may give rise to emotional processing difficulties and hence the symptoms described above. The characteristics that he suggests have a negative influence on emotional processing include the event being sudden, intense, dangerous, uncontrollable, unpredictable and irregular. Most of these factors are present in every violent episode and so would make them particularly difficult to process.

Subjective stimulus factors

In Lazarus and Folkman's (1984) theory of the effects of stress, it is the perception of threat that is the major predictive factor for the severity of psychological reactions, not the actual threat posed. If the victim imagined that it was possible to be killed despite the strong objective evidence to the contrary, then the incident would have a more severe effect, in other words it is the appraisal of the threat that matters.

For people who experience violence at work the perception may be affected further by the assessment of subsequent risk. For health care workers the actual risk of recurrence is relatively high (usually because they have to work with the same or similar patient) and so their appraisal is likely to make the psychological reactions more severe.

A further study by Feinstein and Dolan (1991) investigated whether the actual severity of the event affects the development of long-term difficulties. They looked at people who had fractures of lower limbs which required admission to an orthopaedic ward. Although they only included a few people with assaults, they showed that the factor that best predicted outcome at 6 months was the initial psychological reaction to the injury. This study suggests that it is the way in which the individual assimilates and deals with the traumatic event initially that has the greatest influence on long-term outcome.

Other nonstimulus bound constraints

Psychological reactions are not only affected by what happened during the incident and the subsequent appraisal, they are also certainly affected by the circumstances following it. The responses from colleagues, the employer and likely social supports also have their effects. If there is little social support from friends or the organization, or there is open criticism and blame of the victim then the psychological consequences are likely to be worse.

A direct buffering effect of social support on the effects of psychological problems has not, however, been demonstrated for these sorts of victims. There are several researchers who have proposed that social support is more strongly linked to mental health than physical health (e.g. Ganster and Victor, 1988). This conclusion is based on studies linking psychiatric morbidity and social support after life events. As well as those studies that report a buffering effect of social support (i.e. it reduces the outcome) there are others that show no effects and even some that show a reverse buffering effect (i.e. that people receiving high levels of support also show high levels of psychological difficulties). This reverse buffering effect was found by Whittington and Wykes (1992). They suggested two possible reasons for it: (i) that the quality of the support given was poor, which increased the feelings of helplessness of the victim; or (ii) that social support, which is not easily accessible within a hospital environment, is given to those who are seen to be suffering. In their study, two measures of psychological reactions were collected, one behavioural and the other subjective. A detailed analysis supported the second hypothesis because they found a relationship between the behavioural but not the subjective experiences of psychological distress. In other words, people who showed their distress attracted more social support. However, they also found that most of the social support fell into a category of emotional support, which is thought to assist in the appraisal stage and little informational and instrumental support was given, which is thought to help in the coping phase (Payne and Jones, 1987).

Beliefs

What seems similar across victim categories is the effects on the victim's assumptive world. Janoff-Bulman (1988) suggests that three core assumptions are violated by a threat or attack. These are: (i) the world is benevolent; (ii) events in the world are meaningful; and (iii) the self is positive and worthy. For victims of violence the world is not only a place in which negative events occur but people can no longer be trusted. In trying to answer the question of 'why me?' the victim also has to face the randomness or arbitrariness of the world. This often results in the hypothesis that they have been singled out, which produces thoughts of self-blame and loss of self-esteem.

Abramson *et al.* (1978) have used this cognitive appraisal to make predictions about helpful and unhelpful explanations for uncontrollable aversive events. These explanations contain three dimensions: (i) the source (internal–external); (ii) the generality over time (stable–unstable), and (iii) the generality across situations (specific–unspecific). Victims who attribute the cause of the event to themselves (internal) will experience loss of self-esteem and if they consider the events to be uncontrollable in the future (unstable) and not specific to a particular situation (unspecific) then their symptoms are likely to be more persistent.

Personal and circumstantial characteristics

In trying to distinguish why some individuals develop longer-lasting psychological reactions to events and why some do not, models of PTSD have been proposed, which suggest that the subsequent disorder is a function of pre-existing psychopathology. In other words, the person who develops such reactions had something wrong with them prior to the assault. However, there are few data to support this contention and because of the observed generalized response patterns that seem to be independent of pre-existing personality, this model has few advocates (Boulanger, 1986; Emery *et al.*, 1991). There is some support for the view that personal characteristics that fall within the normal range affect post-traumatic adjustment. Some of these characteristics are the ability to seek support, personal interpretation of events, level of education and psychological role (Green *et al.*, 1985). Unfortunately the definitions of these characteristics are poor.

Personal historical factors such as the level of stress during childhood and previous stressful life events are predisposing factors (Emery *et al.*, 1991). Further support for this model comes from Breslau and colleagues (Breslau *et al.*, 1991) who found that the prevalence of PTSD over a lifetime in a community sample of young adults following a stressful event was 9.2%. They also separated lifestyle factors, which make people more likely to be exposed to a stressor, and the personal predispositions, which affect the likelihood of developing PTSD. The predispositional factors included: (i) being a woman; (ii) a family history of instability; (iii) early separation in childhood; (iv) pre-existing anxiety; and (v) a family history of anxiety. Although this is a cross-sectional study it was free of the contaminating effects of legal and medical interests that bedevil other studies in this area.

SUMMARY

The empirical and theoretical evidence suggests the following:

1. Psychological disabilities including PTSD can occur even when the event is common rather than 'outside the range of human experience'. This then covers the problem that some violence or threats at work are common experiences and even 'daily hassles' (Solomon and Canino, 1989; Breslau and Davis, 1987; Breslau *et al.*, 1991).
2. The long-term outcome is not based on the severity of the injury but is more closely related to the initial psychological reaction (Feinstein and Dolan, 1991).
3. The reaction can be affected by the individual's appraisal of the threat (Abramson *et al.*, 1978; Janoff-Bulman, 1988; Lazarus and Folkman, 1984) and may also be affected by concurrent and previous stressors (Emery *et al.*, 1991).
4. Two theories (Horowitz, 1986; Rachman, 1980) provide a framework for understanding the role of symptoms following stressful responses. Horowitz believes that these are 'normal' responses to abnormal events whereas Rachman suggests that they are signs of poor processing. These might be distinguishable longitudinally. Early signs of intrusive thoughts may be evidence of emotional processing but later signs, especially if they are persistent, may indicate that emotional processing has not achieved a psychological integration of the event. Further longitudinal studies where victims are contacted within a short time of the incident and followed up later, such as that carried out by Wykes (1993), should enable this distinction to be further elaborated.

An integrative model of factors that affect the psychological symptoms

The model shown in Figure 6.1 tries to integrate both the theoretical and practical information reviewed in this chapter. It is provided as a summary and as a suggestion for further research. The interaction

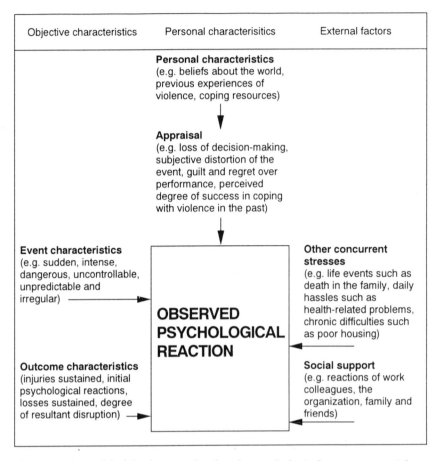

| Objective characteristics | Personal characterisitics | External factors |

Personal characteristics
(e.g. beliefs about the world,
previous experiences of
violence, coping resources)

Appraisal
(e.g. loss of decision-making,
subjective distortion of the
event, guilt and regret over
performance, perceived
degree of success in coping
with violence in the past)

Event characteristics
(e.g. sudden, intense,
dangerous, uncontrollable,
unpredictable and
irregular)

**OBSERVED
PSYCHOLOGICAL
REACTION**

**Other concurrent
stresses**
(e.g. life events such as
death in the family, daily
hassles such as
health-related problems,
chronic difficulties such
as poor housing)

Outcome characteristics
(injuries sustained, initial
psychological reactions,
losses sustained, degree
of resultant disruption)

Social support
(e.g. reactions of work
colleagues, the
organization, family and
friends)

Figure 6.1 A model of the factors related to the psychological responses to violent incidents.

of some factors is not yet clear. For instance, the effects of the objective stimulus measures are not so obvious as they may first appear. The subjects in Lanza's study (Lanza, 1983), reported less fear of the patient the more severely they had been injured. The victims of less serious assaults may be imagining that worse could have happened and that in their imagined event they would not have fared so well. In other words, their appraisal of the event was the most important factor affecting their symptoms.

The aim of this chapter was to categorize some of the responses that victims may experience following an assault. Some explanations of why this should happen and which factors may affect the overall processing of the event were detailed. However, no ways of overcoming or short-circuiting these reactions were described.

This information is given in a further chapter on coping with these responses.

The reason for reviewing the relevant theoretical literature was to dispel the attitude of both employers and employees in the health care field that an individual should be able to withstand the effects of violence: first, because it is part of the job and, second, because there must be something wrong with an individual's coping skills if they experience psychological effects. The research in this area is quite clear. Both objective and subjective factors affect the severity of the psychological reactions. These reactions become more inevitable when the trauma becomes more severe but are nevertheless still possible when the stressors are more 'normal'.

The recognition of the psychopathological effects of violence, especially in the context of work, should enable all who come into contact with the victims of violence to recognize and validate the victim's experiences. This can only lead to a better understanding by organizations and more appropriate support.

REFERENCES

Abramson, L., Seligman, M. and Teasdale, J. (1978) Learned helplessness in humans: Critique and reformulation. *Journal of Abnormal Psychology*, **87**, 49–94.

American Psychiatric Association (1989) *Diagnostic and Statistical Manual of Mental Disorders*, revised 3rd edn, AMA, Washington DC.

Banking and Finance Union (1993) *Armed Robbery: Bank and Building Society Branches. Consultative document by the Health and Safety Executive Financial Services Working Party*.

BASW (1988) *Violence to Social Workers*, British Association of Social Workers, Birmingham.

Boulanger, G. (1986) Predisposition to post-traumatic stress, in *The Vietnam Veteran Redefined* (eds G. Boulanger and C. Kadushin), Lawrence Erlbaum, Hillsdale, New Jersey, pp. 37–50.

Breslau, N. and Davis, G. (1987) Post-traumatic stress disorder: The stressor criterion, *Journal of Nervous and Mental Disease*, **175**, 255–64.

Breslau, N., Davis G., Andreski, P. *et al.* (1991) Traumatic events and post-traumatic stress disorder in an urban population of young adults. *Archives of General Psychiatry*, **48**, 216–22.

Brown, R., Bute, S. and Ford,P. (1986) *Social Workers at Risk. The Management and Prevention of Violence*, Macmillan, Basingstoke.

Burgess, A. and Holmstrom, L. (1974) Rape trauma syndrome. *American Journal of Psychiatry*, **131**, 981–86.

Bute, S.F. (1979) The threat of violence in close encounters with clients, *Social Work Today*, **11**(14), 12–15.

Conn, L. and Lion, J. (1983) Assaults in a university hospital, in *Assaults within Psychiatric Facilities*, (eds J.Lion and W. Reid), W.B. Saunders, Philadelphia, pp. 61–69.

D'Urso, P. and Hobbs, R. (1989) Aggression and the general practitioner. *British Medical Journal*, **298**, 97–8.

Duckworth, D. (1990) *The Nature and Effects of Incidents Which Induce Trauma in Police Officers*. Report to the joint working party on Organisational Health and Welfare, Home Office (ref. SC/86 22/89/1).

Emery, O., Emery, P., Sham, D. *et al*. (1991) Predisposing variables in PTSD patients. *Journal of Traumatic Stress*, **4**, 325–43.

Feinstein, A. and Dolan, R. (1991) Predictors of post-traumatic stress disorder following physical trauma: an examination of the stressor criterion. *Psychological Medicine*, **21** 85–91.

Fisher, N. and Jacoby, R. (1992) Psychiatric morbidity in bus crews following violent assault: a follow-up study. *Psychological Medicine*, **22**, 685–93.

Flannery, R., Fulton, P., Tausch, J. *et al*. (1991) A program to help staff cope with psychological sequelae of assaults by patients. *Hospital and Community Psychiatry*, **42**, 935–38.

Ganster, D. and Victor, B. (1988) The impact of social support on mental and physical health. *British Journal of Medical Psychology*, **61**, 17–36.

Green, B., Wilson, J. and Lindy, J. (1985) Conceptualizing post-traumatic stress disorder, a psychosocial framework, in *Trauma and its Wake: The Study and Treatment of Post-traumatic Stress Disorder*, vol. 1, (ed. C. Figley), Brunner/Mazel, New York, pp. 53–69.

Horowitz, M. (1986) *Stress Response Syndromes*, 2nd edn, Jason Aronson, New York.

Hough, M. and Mayhew, P. (1985) Taking Account of Crime: Key Findings From the Second British Crime Survey, *Home Office Research Study No. 85*, HMSO, London.

Janoff-Bulman, R. (1988) Victims of violence, in *Handbook of Stress, Cognition and Health*, (eds S. Fisher and J. Reason), John Wiley, Chichester.

Kilpatrick, D., Saunders, B., Amick-McMullan, A. *et al*. (1989) Victim and crime factors associated with the development of crime-related post-traumatic stress disorder. *Behavior Therapy*, **20**, 199–214.

Lanza, M. (1983) The reactions of nursing staff to physical assault by a patient. *Hospital and Community Psychiatry*, **34**(1), 44–47.

Lanza, M. (1984) Factors affecting blame placement for patient assault upon nurses. *Issues in Mental Health Nursing*, **6**, 143–61.

Lanza, M. (1987) The relationship between severity of assault to blame placement for assault. *Archives of Psychiatric Nursing*, **1**, 269–79.

Lazarus, R.S. and Folkman, S. (1984) *Stress, Appraisal and Coping*, Springer, New York.

Maguire, M. and Corbett, C. (1987) *The Effects of Crime and the Work of the Victim-support Schemes*, Gower, Aldershot.

Mawby, R. and Gill, M. (1987) *Crime Victims: Needs, Services and the Voluntary Sector*, Tavistock, London.

Payne, R.L. and Jones, J.G. (1987) Measurement and methodology issues in social support, in *Stress and Health: Issues in Research Methodology*, (eds S.V. Kasl and C. Cooper), John Wiley, Chichester.

Poster, E. and Ryan, J. (1989) Nurses' attitudes toward physical assaults by patients. *Archives of Psychiatric Nursing*, **3**, 315–22.

Protheroe, C. (1987) How social workers can cope with being victims. *Social Work Today*, **19**(4), 10–12.

Rachman, S. (1980) Emotional processing. *Behaviour Research and Therapy*, **18**, 51–60.

Rowett, C. (1986) Violence in Social Work. *Institute of Criminology Occasional Paper No. 14*, Cambridge University.

Ryan, J. and Poster, E. (1989) The assaulted nurse: short-term and long-term responses. *Archives of Psychiatric Nursing*, **3**, 323–31.

Shapland, J., Willmore, J. and Duff, P. (1985) *Victims in the Criminal Justice System*, Gower, Aldershot.

Shepherd, J., Qureshi, R., Preston, M. *et al.* (1990) Psychological distress after assaults and accidents. *British Medical Journal*, **301**, 849–50.

Shouksmith, G. and Wallis, D. (1988) Stress amongst hospital nurses, in *Stress and Organisational Problems in Hospitals: Implications for Management*, (eds D. Wallis and C.J. de Wolf), Croom Helm, London.

Solomon, S. and Canino, G. (1989) *Apropriateness of DSM11r Criteria for Post-traumatic Stress Disorder*. Paper presented to the Third International Conference on Traumatic Stress, San Francisco.

Whittington, R. and Wykes, T. (1989) Invisible injury. *Nursing Times*, **85**, 30–32.

Whittington, R. and Wykes, T. (1992) Staff strain and social support in a psychiatric hospital following assault by a patient. *Journal of Advanced Nursing*, **17**, 480–86.

Wykes, T. (1993) *The Psychological Effects of Assault on Nurses: Cognitive Predictors of Outcome*. Paper presented to the third ECOTS Conference, Bergen, June.

CHAPTER 7

Compensation and the criminal justice system

David Miers and Joanna Shapland

INTRODUCTION

A patient runs amok in a hospital or a general practitioner's surgery, he attacks a nurse and some other patients, causing each of them serious personal harm. While, in practice, such incidents are relatively rare (verbal abuse and threats being more common) our concern in this chapter is with what the law has to say on such questions as to whether the patient should be prosecuted and whether the victims can obtain compensation from him or some other source. What if the patient was known by the hospital management or his GP to have violent propensities or suffers from a mental disorder; how do these facts affect the picture?

Health care staff can, of course, be involved with a violent assault in several different roles. They may be the victim of the assault and, possibly, be seeking compensation, or they may themselves be responsible for managing the environment in which the assault occurred. In the latter case, they may need to look at how the incident occurred, the lessons that its occurrence has for a health care setting (e.g. concerning security arrangements) and its effect on staff, including the victim. They may, in addition, be responsible for the staff concerned, with a direct role in supporting them and deciding whether to call the police or other responsible authorities. On the other hand, they may be acting for the health authority or the practice and so represent the body that may be sued by staff, for example, for its failure to maintain a safe system of work. Thus it is quite possible for staff, especially senior staff, to occupy more than one of these roles at once; for example, to be both the victim and responsible for managing the environment in which the assault occurred. In this chapter the relevant legal provisions have been set out in such a way in an attempt to be informative to staff occupying any of these roles. However, it is important to underline that the roles can conflict and at the end of the chapter a few pointers to good practice are offered, which, if adopted, may lessen the problems and hurt that can ensue when something like an assault occurs. The legal remedies discussed relate to England and Wales, although similar possibilities exist in Scotland.

BASIC ISSUES

Crimes and torts: suing the offender

Whenever one person attacks another, the attacker commits both a civil wrong (called a tort) and a crime (unless able to sustain a legally recognized excuse – e.g. such degree of mental disorder as for legal purposes will be treated as lack of capacity – or a justification – e.g. acting in self-defence). It may appear unusual to say of a rapist that he has committed assault and battery against his victim or that a murderer can be sued by the victim's dependants under the Fatal Accidents Act 1976 but, as a matter of legal theory, there is no objection at all.

It is certainly rare for civil proceedings to follow an obviously criminal offence against the person; indeed, there are many reasons why victims might be reluctant to undertake them, such as cost, delay, anxiety and the possibility that the offender may have few resources to meet any award of damages: in short, the disincentives that attach routinely to civil litigation (although some of these may be aggravated precisely because the attack was criminal). Nevertheless, in recent years, there have been instances of women suing men for such crimes as rape and indecent assault (*W. v. Meah*, 1986) and in 1991 Mrs Gail Halford succeeded in obtaining damages against Michael Brookes when the High Court held, notwithstanding that he had not been convicted of the offence, that he had murdered her daughter (*Halford v. Brookes*, 1991).

Indeed, there may be occasions on which it would be more advantageous to sue the offender than seek compensation via the criminal justice system. Two of these concern the grounds upon which compensation may be awarded by the Criminal Injuries Compensation Board (CICB), which is discussed in more detail on page 143. First, the terms under which it operates do not permit it to award compensation for what in the law of damages are called 'aggravated damages'. In *W. v. Meah* (1986), where the defendant viciously raped two women and subjected them to gross indecencies, the High Court was able to award them damages for the aggravated nature of their injuries: however, this was not a factor that the CICB did (or could) take into account when they applied to it for compensation (Miers, 1990, p. 172; Greer, 1991, p. 146).

Second, the CICB is required to take into account the conduct of the victim when it is determining whether to award compensation. It has a wide discretion, which it exercises rigorously. At common law, a person who is injured while committing a criminal offence will not necessarily be precluded from suing the person who caused the injury. For example, in *Lane v. Holloway* (1968), the plaintiff, a 64-year-old man, first addressed his assailant's wife as 'a monkey faced tart' and then took a swing at him. The assailant, who was some 40 years younger, punched the plaintiff in the eye, causing serious injury. Despite his provocative (and unlawful) behaviour, the plaintiff was not barred from suing the younger man. However, had he applied to the CICB for compensation he would almost certainly have been refused. Moreover, the CICB can refuse or reduce compensation where the victim has a criminal record, even though that has no connection with the injury sustained. Here again the common law would be more advantageous as it takes no account of a person's character unless it bears upon the matter in dispute.

A third reason why it might prove more advantageous to sue the offender rather than seek compensation via the criminal justice system concerns the standard of proof affecting the availability of compensation orders. A court can order an offender convicted before it to compensate the victim; such conviction will, of course, be returned only where the prosecution discharges the standard of proof applicable in criminal proceedings, that is, to prove beyond reasonable doubt that the defendant is guilty. However, as Mrs Halford discovered, where a court finds the defendant liable in civil proceedings for the victim's injury, it needs only to be satisfied of his 'guilt' on a balance of probabilities, as it is this lower standard of proof that is applicable in civil law.

Suing a third party

It is always open to a victim of a criminal assault to sue the assailant; it may also be possible for the victim to sue a third party. This latter possibility arises under either or both of two conditions, depending on whether the victim is the third party's employee. Where the victim is an employee, the conditions overlap. First, we comment briefly on the possibility of civil liability being imposed upon hospital authorities (or GPs' practices) for injuries inflicted on their employees during the course of their employment. Second, the question of whether hospital authorities (or GPs' practices) may be liable for injuries caused by one of their patients otherwise than on the basis of their status as employers is considered; in particular, on the basis that they are aware of this patient's violent propensities. Recalling the short set of facts given in the introduction, it can be seen that the nurse may be able to recover on either basis (i.e. as an employee or because the injury was foreseeable) whereas the other patient who was also injured will only be able to recover, if at all, on the second.

Liability based on employment

As a general proposition, employers have a legal duty to provide a safe system of work for their employees (Chapter 1). (Employers may also be vicariously liable for torts committed by their employees in the course of their employment.) This duty may be enforceable by injured employees under any one or more of three legal regimes.

First, it may be a matter covered by the employee's contract of employment. It is not possible to generalize further about contractual remedies here, since liability will depend principally on what the contract specifies.

Second, as MacKay described in Chaper 1, the Health and Safety at Work etc. Act 1974 imposes both general and specific obligations on employers to maintain safe systems of work. This obligation can, in given instances, include taking steps to protect employees so far as is reasonably practicable from the risk of criminal violence by the public (*West Bromwich Building Society v. Townsend*, 1983). Under some circumstances the employer may be liable in tort law for damages for injuries caused to an employee as a result of a breach of these specific statutory duties. It must be noted here that, at the time of writing, violence at work is not legally an accident that has to be reported to the Health and Safety Executive (HSE), and so such incidents will not be investigated by the Factory Inspectorate as accidents at work. However, employers' policies on violence at work can properly be the subject of Factory Inspectors' enquiries when they inspect health care premises (Derrick, 1991) and the HSE has issued guidance to employers as to what should be included in their health and safety policy on violence at work (Health and Safety Executive, 1989).

Third, employers have a common law duty in tort (i.e. apart from their statutory duties under the Health and Safety at Work etc. Act 1974) to take reasonable care to ensure that their employees are, while acting in the course of their employment, not exposed to unnecessary risks, even the risk of being a victim of crime (*Charlton v. Forrest Ink Printing*, 1980). It is rather less easy to point to cases where, despite the employee sustaining a criminal injury, the employer was found to have been in breach of this duty. This is so largely, of course, because most employments do not carry with them the risk of criminal attack upon which the duty to protect the employee would have to be founded. The cases in which the matter has been tested typically arise where employees of security firms and banks sustain injuries in a robbery, or an employee is robbed while on the way to deposit the day's takings from a shop or restaurant in a night safe. In essence, where employers in such cases have taken reasonable care to secure their employees' personal safety from criminal attack there will be no liability. They may do this by providing an escort or, if necessary, secure and reliable motor transport, or they may instruct their employees to vary their route and, if walking, to take a well populated route.

Bearing in mind that in these cases there was *prima facie* the risk of a criminal attack, it is unlikely that a health authority would be held liable in civil proceedings for injuries sustained by its employees at the hands of a person for whom the authority has no responsibility. A health worker who, while at work, is attacked or sexually assaulted by someone visiting a patient, delivering goods to a hospital or other unit, or simply being on the premises for the purpose of committing an offence, will have no remedy against the authority or the general practitioners at whose surgery the incident occurred. The matter may well be different where the offender is a patient (see section on liability to the victim).

RESPONSIBILITY FOR VIOLENT PATIENTS

Suppose that, on the basis of clinical observation, a psychotherapist has reasonable grounds for believing that a patient presents a credible threat of physical danger to another identifiable person. Does the psychotherapist have a legal duty to warn that person, and if no warning is given, may the victim sue the psychotherapist if the threat is realized? These were the questions to which the California Supreme Court gave affirmative answers in *Tarasoff v. Regents of the University of California* (1974). In answering the question whether this also represents the law in England and Wales, two fundamental issues need to be distinguished; that of the practitioner's confidential relationship with the patient and that of his or her liability for injuries attributable to negligent diagnosis or treatment.

Confidentiality

One of the most important aspects of the relationship between a patient and a medical practitioner is the practitioner's duty to treat as confidential matters that pass between them or which otherwise concern the patient. As the GMC's Blue Book puts it:

> It is a doctor's duty ... strictly to observe the rule of professional secrecy by refraining from disclosing voluntarily to any third party information about a patient which he has learnt directly or indirectly in his professional capacity as a registered medical practitioner.

Similarly, the British Psychological Society's Code of Conduct for Psychologists (1985) states:

[Psychologists shall] convey personally identifiable information obtained in the course of professional work to others, only with the expressed permission of those who would be identified ...

There are, however, exceptions to this duty of confidence; thus the question arises, under what circumstances, if any, may the practitioner treating a violent patient disclose to a third party (the police, or the potential victim(s)) the fact of the patient's violent propensities. (This does not concern sharing information with other practitioners having responsibility for the clinical management of the patient; para. 78(b) of the GMC guidelines.) For medical practitioners, of the eight exceptions in the Blue Book, only that contained in para. 78(g) offers any scope for such disclosure. This provides:

rarely, disclosure may be justified on the ground that it is in the public interest, which, in certain circumstances such as, for example, investigation by the police of a grave or very serious crime, might override the doctor's duty to maintain his patient's confidence.

Thus in a case in 1914 it was held that a practitioner would be justified in disclosing to the police information about a patient relevant to the trial for murder of an alleged abortionist, the patient having disclosed the abortionist's identity to her doctor before she died (Mason and McCall Smith, 1991, p. 17). Of more relevance to these issues is the important decision of the Court of Appeal in *W. v. Egdell* (1990).

'W' had been detained as a patient in a secure special hospital under a restriction order (without limit of time) following his conviction for manslaughter on the grounds of diminished responsibility. He had shot and killed five people, and caused injury to others by means of homemade bombs. He had been diagnosed as suffering from paranoid schizophrenia. Ten years later he applied for a transfer to another hospital (ultimately with a view to being returned to the community). In his report for the Mental Health Review Tribunal, his responsible medical officer, a consultant psychiatrist, recommended that provided he remained on medication, W no longer presented a danger to the public. W's solicitors also sought an independent assessment from another consultant, Dr Egdell, but his opinion differed markedly from this recommendation. In his judgment W's condition was more serious (he still showed interest in homemade bombs) and was not yet amenable to medication. Coupled with his other observations of W's case, Dr Egdell concluded that it would not be safe to release him from custody.

In view of this, W's application was withdrawn; but when his case came up for routine consideration by the Tribunal some time later,

Dr Egdell discovered that his report had not been (as W's solicitors' letter had implied it would be) forwarded either to the Tribunal or to the hospital. He then sought the solicitors' agreement that it should be. When this was refused on W's instructions, he himself sent a copy to the hospital, urging that a copy also be sent to the Home Secretary. In the subsequent litigation the question naturally arose whether Dr Egdell had acted in the public interest when he broke his confidence with W. Both the High Court and the Court of Appeal held that he had. Bingham LJ said:

> Where a man has committed multiple killings under the disability of serious mental illness, decisions that may lead directly or indirectly to his release from hospital should not be taken unless the responsible authority is properly able to make an informed judgment that the risk of repetition is so small as to be acceptable. A consultant psychiatrist who becomes aware, even in the course of a confidential relationship, of information which leads him, in the exercise of what the court considers a sound professional judgment, to fear that such decisions may be made on inadequate information and with a real risk of consequent danger to the public is entitled to take such steps as are reasonable in all the circumstances to communicate the grounds of his concern to the responsible authorities.
>
> (*W. v. Egdell*, 1990)

How wide a discretion does this, 'the most nebulous of all the exceptions' (Jones, 1990, p. 17), thus permit the practitioner to disclose confidential material? Central to the decisions of both courts were the particular circumstances of W's detention and of the commissioning of Dr Egdell's report. W was not an ordinary member of the public; his release from detention was dependent upon the psychiatric judgment that he no longer posed a threat. Dr Egdell therefore owed a duty not only to W but to the public; the question that he was being asked to address was exactly whether it was in the public interest that W should be released. In the instant case 'the fear of a real risk to public safety entitled [the] doctor to take reasonable steps to communicate the ground of his concern to the appropriate authorities' (Mason and McCall Smith, 1991, p. 179; *R. v. Crozier*, 1990); but only the most compelling circumstances can justify such disclosure, since it is also in the public interest that patients retain confidence in the confidentiality of the medical advice they seek.

Two variations upon this case may now be considered. Suppose, first, that the patient did not have W's institutional history, but was instead seeking psychiatric counselling for sexual difficulties and presented in a manner that was consistent with the commission of a series of sexual offences, which, to the psychiatrist's knowledge, the police were investigating. If, in the doctor's professional judgment there is a real risk of injury to a member of the public (*a fortiori* where, as in *Tarasoff v. Regents of the University of California* (1974), the patient identifies a person whom he or she intends to harm), *W. v. Egdell* indicates that it will be in the public interest to disclose this information, at least to the police. Thus the practitioner would have a good answer to any complaint about the disclosure made before a court of law or a disciplinary body.

Other professions' codes of practice may have slightly differently worded exceptions to the general rule relating to confidentiality. So, for example, the British Psychological Society's Code of Conduct contains the provision that psychologists shall:

> in exceptional circumstances, where there is sufficient evidence to raise serious concern about the safety or interests of recipients of services, or about others who may be threatened by the recipient's behaviour, take such steps as are judged necessary to inform appropriate third parties without prior consent after first consulting an experienced and disinterested colleague, unless the delay caused by seeking this advice would involve a significant risk of life or health.
>
> (*British Psychological Society, 1985*)

However, it is not clear how the courts will interpret the legal liability of psychologists or other nonmedical practitioners.

The second variation may be posed as follows. Suppose that Dr Egdell had not disclosed his report to the hospital, that W had been transferred and eventually released from custody and had then killed. Would the victim's dependants be able to sue Dr Egdell? In other words, is there not merely a discretion to disclose but also a duty of care, as *Tarasoff* indicated, to potential victims?

Liability for injury

So far as liability is concerned, the primary issue of concern is the liability of the practitioner to the violent patient's victim(s). However, it should also be borne in mind that the practitioner may be liable **to the patient** should it be proven, for example, that the treatment that was prescribed was ill-advised or that the patient was released prematurely, in consequence of which the patient has now been convicted of an offence against the person. This issue goes beyond the scope of this chapter and is not dealt with here. So far as legal principles apply, they would be the normal principles of the law of negligence, since *prima facie* the authority owes a duty of care to those whom it is treating (*Barnett v. Chelsea and Kensington Hospital Management Committee*, 1969).

Liability to the victim

In this section we consider whether practitioners owe a duty of care to health workers and other potential victims when they are treating patients known to them to be violent. As has been indicated, if liability arises here it does so independently of any legal relationship of employment between the defendant and the victim; however, as we shall see, the fact that a health worker is employed by the defendant may be relevant in determining whether such a special relationship exists between the defendant and the victim as gives rise to a duty of care in tort.

If the practitioner is to be liable, a necessary condition is that, given the facts, he or she owed a duty of care to the particular victim. It will also be necessary to show that the practitioner was in breach of the duty, and that the breach caused (both as a matter of law and of fact) the injury; put in other terms, the fact that a practitioner owes a duty of care does not necessarily mean that there will be liability even if a person sustains an injury. The law of negligence requires that the injury to the victim was foreseeable, that the victim was in a sufficiently proximate relationship with the negligent practitioner (or authority) and that it would be just and reasonable to impose a duty of care. This proposition was confirmed in 1989 in *Hill v. Chief Constable for West Yorkshire* (1989), litigation that arose from the failure of the West Yorkshire police to capture Peter Sutcliffe ('the Yorkshire Ripper') who, over a 5-year period, committed 13 murders and eight attempted murders. The House of Lords rejected the claim by the mother of his last victim that the police had, through their failure to test and to attend properly to the evidence they had accumulated, been negligent with regard to her daughter's safety. In the absence of any special relationship between the victim and the police over and above the normal requirement for liability in negligence that harm to a victim be reasonably foreseeable, the House held that although injury to women of the class represented by Sutcliffe's victims was foreseeable, this victim was not in a sufficiently proximate relationship with the police. According to the House of Lords' earlier decision, *Home Office v. Dorset Yacht Co.* (1970), proximity arose either where the person causing the damage (or injury) had been under the defendant's supervision and control, or where the proximity or identity of the plaintiff made damage (or injury) very likely. In either case, the defendant *prima facie* owes a duty of care to safeguard the victim from the offender's actions. In this case the Home Office was, through its responsibilities for borstal arrangements, liable when some Borstal boys escaped the negligent custody of their officers, boarded a yacht and caused damage both to it and to another yacht.

The potential application of this principle to violent patients is obvious. First, where a patient is known to be violent and is under the supervision and control of the practitioner (or the appropriate authority), in circumstances in which it is foreseeable that the patient will cause injury should he or she escape, there is a strong argument that a duty of care will be owed to the victim. The extent of any liability based on this principle will of course depend on the exact facts. In litigation arising from injuries inflicted by one prisoner upon another, the courts have, while agreeing that the prison authorities owe a duty of care to protect one prisoner from another (*Ellis v. Home Office*, 1953), in most cases found the Home Office not to be liable. This has been so because on the facts of each case, it was found that the authorities had no reason to know that the assailant was any more violent than any other prisoner, that they had taken reasonable care to supply sufficient staff to protect prisoners, or that the assault was spontaneous and could not reasonably have been foreseen by an experienced officer. On the other hand, if the prison (or the hospital) authority had not taken reasonable care in the circumstances, liability could follow. So in *Holgate v. Lancashire Mental Hospitals Board* (1937) it was held that a hospital authority was liable when it negligently released on licence a violent patient who was being compulsorily detained and who then attacked the plaintiff. It must be emphasized that the issue of liability in such cases is complex,* although a health authority may be prepared to make a compensatory payment while rejecting legal responsibility for the injury.†

Second, liability may exist where there is a sufficient degree of proximity between the practitioner and the victim. If the victim is but 'one of a vast number of potential victims at risk' (*Hill v. Chief Constable for West Yorkshire*, 1989, p. 62), then, in the absence of any other consideration, there will be no duty of care. However, if the victim, although not individually identifiable, is a member of a narrow class of potential victims, there may at least, as the Ontario High Court held in *Doe v. Board of Commissioners of Police for Metropolitan Toronto* (1989), be a triable issue. Here the police investigating a

---

* In *P and others v. Harrow London Borough Council* (1992) the High Court held that boys who had been placed in special schools and who had there suffered sexual abuse by the headmaster were not in a sufficiently proximate relationship with the Local Education Authority to found an action in negligence; neither was the abuse foreseeable in the absence of any knowledge on the LEA's part of the headmaster's proclivities. In August 1992, a teacher commenced proceedings in negligence against her employer for the injuries she received at the hands of a pupil at her school whose history of violent behaviour she alleged was known by the employer.

† In 1992 a health authority paid an undisclosed sum to the parents of a girl stabbed to death by a psychiatric patient who had been released from its control in consequence of a 'serious error of professional judgment', but without accepting legal liability (*The Times*, 17 April 1992).

sequence of rapes had not issued warnings to potential victims, of which the plaintiff was one, because they thought that such warnings would cause panic and would impede the investigation. The plaintiff shared the characteristics of those women who had been raped (e.g. was single, white, living on the 2nd or 3rd floor of an apartment block within a very limited and defined area of Toronto) and was herself raped in her own apartment by the man subsequently convicted of several similar offences. The court held that where there were specific potential victims known to the police (such as passengers on an aircraft suspected of having a bomb planted on it), there was a sufficient proximity between the plaintiff and defendant. Here 'the elements of knowledge, foreseeability and special relationship of proximity' (p. 426), *prima facie* created a duty of care. Thus where the patient is privately consulting a psychiatrist who thereby learns of the identity of a small class of potential victims then, on the basis of the characterization of the special relationship in the *Home Office v. Dorset Yacht Co.* case, it could be argued that having specific knowledge (or an informed opinion about) the likelihood of the patient's offending (that is, the foreseeability of injury), those victims would be sufficiently proximate as to satisfy the second requirement for a duty of care (*a fortiori* if the patient is also under the practitioner's supervision and control).

Nevertheless, whether proximity were based on the relationship between the practitioner and the offender/patient on the one hand, or the victim on the other, a court would also have to conclude that it was just and reasonable to impose such a duty (*Caparo Industries plc v. Dickman*, 1990). In *Hill v. Chief Constable of West Yorkshire* (1989), the House of Lords also said that even if there had been sufficient proximity between Jacqueline Hill and the police, the fact that the imposition of a duty of care would be likely to lead to the adoption by the police of unduly defensive practices so as to avoid claims for negligence itself militated against such imposition. Defensive medicine, like defensive policing, can have a detrimental effect on the performance of professional duties, and thus the courts may take the view, as a matter of public policy, that it will only be in cases where the foresight of injury is very great and the proximity between the victim and the practitioner very close that a duty of care should be imposed.

What then of the charge nurse who is assaulted by a drunk awaiting attention in a busy accident and emergency department on a Friday night? Whether the authority owes the staff a duty of care will depend initially, as we have seen, upon the foreseeability of injury to nurses and others working in that department given the circumstances that normally prevail on a Friday night. As with many questions of liability, it depends, in short, on the facts. If such incidents are common and the authority is fully aware of them and has taken no steps at all to safeguard its employees' personal safety (e.g. by employing security guards to patrol the hospital grounds, by having a guard on duty in casualty, by issuing all staff with personal alarms), a court could well find for the victim employee in a negligence action if there is sufficient proximity between the staff and the authority (highly likely) and it is just and reasonable to impose a duty.

The legal duty of health care workers in relation to information they have about someone in their care who may be about to commit an assault against someone else has been discussed. It must be stressed that this legal duty does not necessarily correspond to the **professional** duty set out in the relevant codes of ethics of the professions or, indeed, the **moral** duty or moral views that any individual may hold.

THE PROSECUTION OF VIOLENT PATIENTS

Criminal prosecutions for most offences other than nonserious motoring offences to which the driver pleads guilty are conducted by the Crown Prosecution Service (CPS). It can only act in response to the institution of criminal proceedings, and this is almost always the consequence of a police decision to charge a suspect with an offence. Accordingly, in determining whether a violent patient who has caused injury (whether to a health care worker or other victim) is likely to be prosecuted, one should begin by considering whether the incident will be reported and how the police are likely to react to the report of an assault. Let us, by way of illustration, first consider this in connection with a simple case in which a patient who is neither intoxicated nor mentally disordered violently attacks a health care worker in the presence of witnesses, causing serious bodily harm.

The simple case

The police are able to investigate any offence, including obviously an assault or a threat of violence. However, in general, they will not investigate offences that have been reported to them by the victim or someone acting on the victim's behalf, unless the offence is serious. Before it is possible to consider the likelihood of a prosecution being mounted, therefore, one needs to see how violent offences in health care settings will be reported to the police.

It is preferable that the institution should have a clear policy about what kinds of offences should be reported to the police and who should take that responsibility and subsequently liaise with the police. When a violent offence has occurred, people will be in some shock and it is unfair to expect those immediately in charge of the situation to be able to take those decisions without any previous consideration. Should there be any chance of the incident being reported it is also important that any evidence of the offence (e.g. a weapon) is left undisturbed. An institutional policy about reporting may differentiate between assaults by staff, patients or outsiders, or according to the situation in which the assault occurred. It is clearly desirable that staff should be informed about such policy, so that they know what action will take place. It is also important to bear in mind that, if the incident is not reported to the police, this may jeopardize a victim's claim for compensation to the Criminal Injuries Compensation Board – although the victim's own responsibility is only to ensure that the incident is reported to the police (if at all possible) or to the competent authority (and not to ensure that the institution reports it). An individual victim can decide to report the incident to the police, even if the institution decides not to – and this could not be held to be in breach of their contract of employment (although the institution might exert some informal pressure on individuals to follow its policy).

It should be noted that reporting to the police does not automatically imply that any prosecution or any particular further action will follow – this will depend on several factors of which the views of the victim and other professionals involved in that health care setting will be significant (although the ultimate decision on action such as arrest or charge remains that of the police).

The decision whether or not to report can be a very difficult one. Even in our 'simple' example, it is not always clear what will be in the patient's best interests, and both legal and health care professionals often disagree among themselves on individual cases. Is it, for example, better not to involve the police at all, in the hope that the patient will not be dragged through the courts? Or would this be paternalistic, denying patients their 'right' to be responsible and to be held to be responsible for their own actions? If informal action is to be taken within the institution, should the matter be investigated by outside professionals to ensure the patient really was the one responsible? The victim's interests may range from a desire to see the offender convicted and ordered to compensate for the injury to a wish to let the matter rest. Moreover, there is an understandable desire of the institution to be seen to be able to manage its own environment in an effective manner. It is in this situation that the different potential roles of professionals can conflict – and where it becomes vital for each person involved to be able to separate out their roles, and to know the policy of the institution.

Whether the police respond to the report of a crime (by the victim or a witness), and what resources they are prepared to allocate to its investigation is entirely a matter for them. The police cannot be compelled as a matter of law to pursue any particular offence notified to them. However, in the illustrative case, at least two of the primary criteria that the police employ when deciding whether to pursue the offence will be met. These are that there has been personal injury to an identifiable victim and that the incident was seen by several witnesses.

One of the options open to the police once they have completed their enquiries is to caution the offender. Revised guidelines published in 1990 (Home Office, 1990a) recommend this course where the offender is a juvenile or is a first offender, and its use requires that the offender admit his guilt. The circular recommends that the victim is consulted before any decision to caution or prosecute is taken – but the police are not bound to follow the victim's wishes. However, it would be unlikely that the police would caution a violent patient where the victim sustained serious personal injury, although they might decide to take no further action where the patient is already undergoing treatment that is likely to minimize the risk of further violence.

On the assumption that the police charge the patient with an offence (typically under sections 18, 20 or 47 of the Offences Against the Person Act 1861), the papers are forwarded to the CPS for prosecution. Like the police, the CPS cannot be compelled in law to act; should it decide not to proceed, the only option is for the victim to prosecute the patient. This is not an easy course; the victim will *prima facie* bear the costs of the prosecution, and neither the police nor the CPS can be compelled in law to hand over the witness statements and other documents relating to the offence that they have in their possession.

In determining whether to prosecute any offence, the CPS is required to have regard to two matters. First it must be satisfied that 'there is admissible, substantial and reliable evidence that a criminal offence known to the law has been committed by an identifiable person' (Code for Crown Prosecutors, 1992). In answering the question of whether there is sufficient evidence of the alleged offence the CPS will look closely at the strength of the evidence and the credibility of the witnesses. Where these witnesses are other health care staff, a prosecution will, given their general credibility with magistrates and juries, more likely than not be pursued. On the other hand, where the assault took place in poor light and the only witness was at a distance, some other convincing evidence will be required. Like the police, the CPS have finite resources and necessarily have to allocate them to stronger rather than weaker cases; as common sense would suggest, the CPS is more likely to prosecute a case with a realistic prospect of conviction than one whose evidence is shaky.

The second matter is whether the prosecution is in the public interest. For example, there may be wholly convincing evidence that an elderly person has stolen some goods from a supermarket but it would almost certainly not be in the public interest to prosecute if

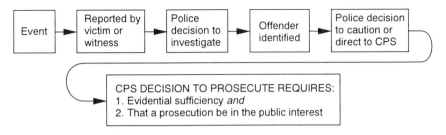

Figure 7.1 The sequence of decisions leading to prosecution of a violent offender.

it transpired that the alleged offender is suffering from Alzheimer's disease. Other factors to which the CPS must have regard are the victim's attitude and the likely penalty. As has been suggested, other things being equal, the more serious the personal injury inflicted by the offender, the greater the public interest in a prosecution.

Presented as a flow chart, the sequence of decisions discussed in this section is shown in Figure 7.1. It should also be clear from what has been said that the rate of attrition in this sequence is considerable.

The disordered and the disorderly patient

Now suppose that the violent patient was intoxicated at the time of the assault, or is suffering from a mental disorder within the meaning of the Mental Health Act 1983. In considering how these variations affect the procedures outlined in the simple case, intoxication will be discussed first.

The violent, intoxicated patient

The basic position that the law adopts is that the fact of voluntary intoxication (whether through alcohol or the use of drugs which it is unlawful for the offender to have in his possession, or through a mixture of alcohol and of drugs which it is lawful for him to have in his possession) is no defence to a criminal charge. The drunk patient who lashes out and hits the victim and then says in court 'I wouldn't have done this if I'd been sober' will merely find the punishment imposed will be more severe. It is, of course, itself a criminal offence to be drunk in a public place.

However, voluntary intoxication may be relevant to the prospects of conviction in two instances. The first is where the offence charged requires that the prosecution prove that the patient **intended** to bring about some prohibited consequence, not that he or she was merely reckless with regard to it. If an intoxicated patient strikes a blow that results in grievous bodily harm, there can be criminal liability under section 20 of the Offences Against the Person Act, 1861, if it can be shown that the patient was, while drunk, acting recklessly. However, if the prosecution is brought under section 18 of that Act (a more serious offence), it will have to be shown that the patient intended to cause that level of injury, and in this case the intoxication may be an obstacle.

The second instance is where the intoxication is diagnosable as a symptom of alcoholism. As this is a matter that relates directly to the patient's mental health, this will be discussed under the next heading.

The mentally disordered patient

As indicated earlier, one of the factors that the CPS has to consider when determining whether it is in the public interest to continue with criminal proceedings is their impact on the alleged offender's mental health (Hoggett, 1990, Chapter 5). Where the CPS is satisfied that the probable adverse effects of a prosecution outweigh the interests of justice, proceedings should be discontinued. Many of the considerations that are relevant to the simple case are aggravated here, though evidence from the USA of the impact on psychiatric patients of criminal proceedings for assaulting hospital staff is conflicting (Hoge and Gutheil, 1987; Miller and Maier, 1987).

Similarly, the police are required to consider carefully whether any formal action is necessary where a suspect appears to be mentally disordered. If the suspect is able to meet the criteria, a caution may be in order. In 1990, the Home Office issued new guidelines intended to encourage the diversion of mentally disordered suspects from the criminal justice system (Home Office, 1990b; Fennell, 1991). These remind the police that they have a duty under the Police and Criminal Evidence Act 1984 to call a police surgeon to the station if a person being detained there (or being brought in) appears to be mentally disordered, and that they should consult the CPS about what further action should be taken. Although the guidelines do not expressly say so, this must apply particularly where the suspect has committed violent assaults on identifiable victims. The police are unlikely to recommend prosecution where the offender is undergoing or is about to undergo compulsory or voluntary treatment as an inpatient and assaults an outsider or member of his or her family (Ashworth and Shapland, 1980); however, it is not clear what their policy is in relation to assaults taking place in hospitals or other health care settings.

Even where the CPS considers it to be in the public interest to prosecute a violent, mentally disordered suspect, it may be, in a few cases, that the person charged is unfit to stand trial or will have a defence of legal insanity. However, these are rare cases,* and where the accused has caused serious injury or death, a prosecution will almost certainly be maintained, even if, as in the case of a prosecution for murder, the result is a conviction for manslaughter on the grounds of diminished responsibility. Among other conditions, the 'abnormality of mind' required by section 2 of the Homicide Act, 1957, may include a person who has clinical alcoholism.

COMPENSATION THROUGH THE CRIMINAL JUSTICE SYSTEM

There are two avenues by which health care staff may be able to obtain compensation through the criminal justice system in the event that they are injured by a violent patient. The first is called a compensation order, the second is through the Criminal Injuries Compensation Board (CICB).

Compensation orders

The scope of compensation orders

The law governing compensation orders (COs) in England and Wales is to be found in sections 35–38 of the Powers of Criminal Courts Act, 1973. Similar provisions exist for Scotland. The 1973 Act permits a court to impose an order upon a person convicted before it, requiring the payment of compensation to anyone who sustained any personal injury, loss or damage as a result of the offence (or of one taken into consideration). A CO is not payable where the offender has been cautioned. COs thus extend both to personal injury and to property loss or damage, and are payable not just to the complainant (although he or she will be the most likely recipient) but, as section 35 says, to anyone who suffered as a result.

Before making an order the court must take the offender's means into account, and must have a sufficiently accurate account of the victim's losses to be able to make an order for a specific sum. In the case of a magistrates' court, this may not exceed £5000; there is no limit in the Crown Court. The order may be payable as a lump sum or in instalments over not more than about 3 years. It may be combined with an immediate custodial sentence, so long as the offender

---

* They may become less rare consequent upon the coming into force of the Criminal Procedure (Insanity and Unfitness to Plead) Act 1991 which removes the previous automatic consequence of the special verdict or a finding of unfitness, that the defendant be committed to a hospital under a restriction order without restriction of time.

has the means to pay and will not be driven to re-offend upon release in order to comply. If the court also wishes to fine the offender, or to make a confiscation order, but the offender has insufficient means to comply with both the CO and the other order, the CO has statutory priority. By agreement between the Lord Chancellor's Department and the CPS, a CO has priority over an order for costs. Where ordered, compensation can be intended to cover both the specific losses incurred by the victim (typically loss of earnings and expenses associated with obtaining medical treatment).

An important development was the imposition by section 104 of the Criminal Justice Act, 1988, of a duty on the court to give reasons why it has not made a CO in a case in which it has power to do so. If a magistrates' court fails to give reasons, the victim can appeal.

Obtaining compensation

A CO offers a realistic prospect of compensation for the injured health care worker only if several conditions are met. First, and most obvious, the patient must be convicted of an offence. If the violent patient is mentally disordered and is diverted from the criminal justice system or is acquitted of the offence, there can be no order. Nor, even in the case of conviction, is an order likely in such cases.

Second, the court will require evidence of the victim's injury. Although the court has a duty to give reasons why it has not made an order in a case in which it has power to make one, its duty does not extend to chasing the victim for information. In theory it should have such information before it if the police/CPS are meeting the advice given by the Home Office to encourage the victim to complete a 'compensation schedule'. This schedule asks for details of any injury, loss or damage, and is intended to be presented to the court at the sentencing stage. The guidelines on this are set out in Home Office circular No. 20/1988 (Home Office, 1988), and if the victim gets in touch with the local branch of *Victim Support* (the national address is given in Appendix A), there ought to be no reason why the schedule is not completed.

The third condition is that the offender has the means to pay a CO. The court has a statutory duty to take this into account before making an order. If the offender indicates that he is willing and able to pay, the court should inquire what sums he can afford to pay, and what the sources are. If it appears that he has a capital asset – a car perhaps – there is no objection to the court making an order on the basis that he sells it, provided that the court can place a value on it. Even if he is unemployed, an offender on income support can be expected to pay up to £5.00 a week in instalments.

The fourth condition concerns the 'value' of the injury sustained. Magistrates can no longer refuse to make an order on the ground that they have no guidelines; a Home Office circular (Home Office, 1988) contains a tariff prepared by the Criminal Injuries Compensation Board (CICB) for specimen injuries. However, they must have the details of the injury: magistrates are quite entitled to refuse to make an award if they cannot establish to their satisfaction the kind of injury sustained.

Success rates

No amount of circulars will improve the victim's position if magistrates' attitudes to compensation are as ambivalent as was revealed in Home Office studies in 1988 (Newburn, 1988) and 1992 (Moxon *et al.*, 1992). These show that while many magistrates express themselves to be in favour of redressing the balance, of making the offender pay, they feel uncomfortable about the need also to punish the offender.

In 1991, 113 000 COs were made, 103 000 by magistrates and 10 000 by the Crown Court (Home Office, 1993). In the case of indictable offences of violence against the person, 19 300 COs were made by magistrates upon summary conviction (58% of all offenders sentenced for this offence) and 3500 were made by the Crown Court (25% of all offenders sentenced). For sexual offences, 200 COs were made following summary conviction (10% of all offenders sentenced), and less than 100 were made by the Crown Court.

Although one must be careful about average figures, the average amount ordered to be paid by magistrates in the case of violence against the person was £125 and, in the case of sexual offences, £105. In the Crown Court, these amounts were £318 and £247 respectively. By comparison, the highest average figure in the magistrates' court for any one offence was £225 (theft and handling) and the average for all offences was £161; in the Crown Court these averages were £2981 (fraud) and £882 respectively.

The figures for personal injury are very low by comparison with the kind of awards routinely made by the CICB. Nevertheless, even if the average figure in a magistrates' court (£125) was an amount payable only in respect of pain and suffering, it is an amount commensurate with virtually the lowest figure on the Home Office's recommended tariff, payable in respect of a black eye (£100) or a minor cut (£75–£200). As it is unlikely that all 19 300 victims sustained only such minor injury, the primary reason for these low figures is almost certainly that, in most cases, the court considered that this was all the offender could afford, irrespective of the tariff value of the injury.

In short, a CO is unlikely to prove an effective source of compensation, in the sense of producing the full monetary value the civil courts or CICB might order, except in cases where the injury caused was relatively minor and the offender obviously has the means to pay. Conversely, COs are part (or the whole) of the sentence of the offender. Many victims feel that compensation should form part of a sentence and see COs as playing an important part of what they believe should happen as the result of the offence (Shapland *et al.*, 1985; Newburn and de Peyrecave, 1987). COs may therefore have symbolic importance for the victim unrelated to the actual monetary value of the award.

The Criminal Injuries Compensation Board (CICB)

The scope of the scheme

The CICB administers a nonstatutory scheme whose latest major revisions came into force on 1 February 1990. It covers England, Wales and Scotland. With one exception, the scheme only applies to personal injuries. The exception is that compensation can be awarded to repair or replace such personal property as spectacles, dentures and hearing aids that are damaged or destroyed in the assault. The personal injuries with which the CICB typically deals arise from the commission of a crime of violence (which includes arson and poisoning); however, the scheme specifies two further types of criminal injury: (i) those arising from law enforcement activity; and (ii) from trespass on a railway. This last is intended to bring within its scope railway employees who suffer trauma from witnessing people committing suicide under trains. So far as health care workers dealing with violent patients are concerned, any claims they make will almost always fall under the category 'crime of violence'; however, it is possible that a worker could suffer physical harm while going to the assistance of a police officer trying to restrain the patient who is making a disturbance in an accident and emergency department, or suffer mental harm should a violent patient seek to injure himself by attempting suicide on a railway track.

Unquestionably one of the most important features of the scheme is that there is no requirement that there be a conviction of the patient (or indeed that the offender be apprehended or even identified). This is clearly of importance where the patient is mentally disordered. There is scant precedent on the question whether a mentally disordered defendant is liable in tort law for the injuries he or she has caused. It is no defence to an action based on assault or battery that the defendant did not know that what he or she was doing was wrong, unless it is proven that the defendant's condition prevented him or her from forming the intention to make contact with the victim. However, the terms of the scheme render such questions unimportant for most, if not all cases in which a health care worker is injured by a disturbed patient. Indeed, the CICB receives a regular number of claims from health care workers injured by geriatric patients or by patients incapable of controlling their bodily movements. Provided that the CICB is satisfied on a balance of probabilities that, had the patient been of sound mind and aware of what was happening, the requirements of a crime of violence (or one of the other categories within the scheme) are met, the claimant will come within its terms.

While no conviction is necessary, it is essential that the victim personally reports the incident giving rise to the injury to the police without delay (unless there is any good reason why the victim is unable to do so). Any claim must be made within 3 years of the incident, and the injury has to be worth more than £1000 (since 6 January 1992) after the deduction of any social security benefits payable. That figure can be arrived at by aggregating the victim's special damages (loss of earnings, medical expenses) and general damages (pain and suffering, loss of amenity) and deducting such state payments as income support or unemployment benefit; however, if the product does not exceed the lower limit, no compensation at all will be payable. The Board also has jurisdiction to refuse or reduce an award because of the conduct of the claimant before, during or after the incident, or because of his character as evidenced by his criminal convictions or unlawful conduct.

Where compensation is payable, it covers both special damages (e.g. loss of earnings and expenditure incurred as a result of the injury) and general damages (i.e. for the pain and suffering caused, which may include mental as well as physical hurt). The figures for general damages are based on common law damages, and therefore can (subject to the deduction rules) be very substantial where the injury is, for example, disabling.

Obtaining compensation

On the assumption that the victim can meet the conditions set out in the preceding section, the single most frustrating feature of the scheme is the delay that attends the resolution of claims: 73% of claims take more than 9 months to resolve; 57% take more than 12 months (Criminal Injuries Compensation Board, 1992). There has been some improvement in the waiting time over the past 2 years in consequence of an increase in the Board's staff and of the introduction in 1990 of new procedures for dealing with claims, but it is bound to take a few more years before the delay ameliorates to something like the position in 1986/87, when 50% of claims were resolved within 9 months.

As with COs, information about the possibility of claiming compensation can be obtained from *Victim Support*; alternatively, the claimant should write to the national office of the CICB (Appendix A).

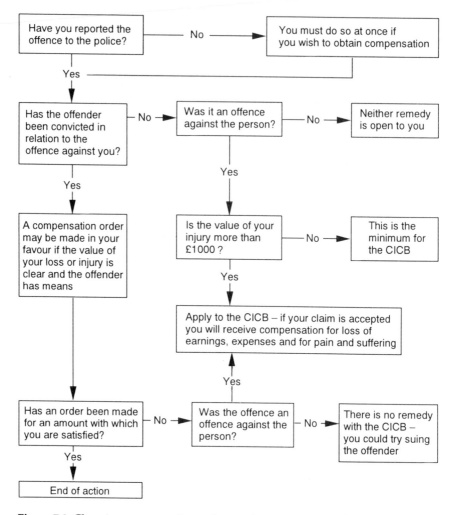

Figure 7.2 Choosing compensation orders or claims to the CICB following a violent incident.

Success rates

In 1991–1992 the Board received 61 400 claims for compensation. Although there is no correlation between that figure and the number of claims resolved in any one year, in the same year the Board made 32 249 awards and refused compensation to 18 256 claimants, while 2608 claims were abandoned. Over the lifetime of the Board, 60–65% of claimants have been successful.

The sums awarded are substantial, following the common law's valuation of injuries. Of course, the value of awards made depends on the severity of the injuries to be compensated, but in 1991–1992 more than 68% of awards exceeded £1000 (Criminal Injuries Compensation Board, 1992, para. 8.2). Figure 7.2 shows the various routes for obtaining compensation.

CONFLICTING ROLES AND GOOD PRACTICE

A violent assault or threat of violence is disturbance enough in a health care setting. The prospect of becoming involved with the legal system tends to be outside the routine experience of many health care professionals and adds to the sense of concern and worry (even panic) that people feel when such an incident occurs. In this chapter, the legal basis of the various options and remedies that may exist and a brief summary of current practice have been described. However, if health care institutions and professionals give some consideration to what might occur and how they would deal with it **before an incident happens**, many of the most distressing effects and consequences can be minimized. If something then does occur, people's reactions as to whether the procedures were helpful can be used to make the procedures better for the future. So, if an incident occurs:

1. Staff need to know to whom it should be reported within the health care setting; that person, in turn, should be given guidance on the circumstances in which external bodies (such as the police) should be called in. The lines of authority and the conditions governing the exercise of any discretion should be clearly spelled out to those who will have the responsibility for its exercise. A member of staff acting in accordance with these guidelines should not be criticized, for example, for calling in an external body.
2. People should be aware what immediate steps should be taken to protect the victim, to control any offender and to 'preserve the scene' of the offence (i.e. to preserve any evidence and account for it).
3. There should be an effective system for keeping records of all violent incidents. This is so that the institution is aware of when and in what circumstances such incidents occur, so it can assess what preventive measures are necessary. This is the cornerstone of the advice given by the Health and Safety Executive on violence at work and is clearly vital to putting together an effective health and safety policy. The HSE issues a free leaflet *Violence to Staff* (1989), which defines what might be considered a violent incident and gives practical and helpful advice for employers and employees. Some case histories of how to set up a good preventive policy are given in Poyner and Warne (1988).

4. Those in charge of the situation must be responsible for assessing what is needed to support the victim and others working in that situation. Remember that the effects of assaults at work can be some of the more severe and more long-lasting effects of violent crime (Shapland *et al.*, 1985) and that they can affect not just the direct victim but others working there. A 'debriefing' session soon after the assault in which people can talk out their reactions in a nonjudgmental atmosphere can be very helpful but there must be no comebacks from what is said then. The institution should have a policy of supporting staff and colleagues involved in violent incidents, which should cover both immediate and more long-term help, including the possibility of referral for counselling or psychiatric or psychological help where this is necessary, and support for managers themselves. The policy should be known to all staff and managers trained to implement it.
5. Staff should be able to obtain information easily about possibilities for compensation, and whether the institution carries personal injury insurance for staff.
6. When taking decisions about reporting, prosecution, compensation and what measures should be taken to prevent similar incidents in the future, it is important to recognize that staff may have to occupy different roles, as set out at the beginning of this chapter. Someone who is a victim but who is also responsible for the management of the facility or area in which the incident occurred may be in the strange position of blaming himself or herself for not preventing the incident, or for inadequate after-care. The sense of guilt and blame that all victims suffer (for somehow having 'caused' the incident) is likely to be several times magnified, particularly if they feel that they have to carry on without showing any effects. It is important for both management and colleagues to be sensitive to this.

In essence, it is in its response to a crisis, such as a violent incident, by which an institution tends to be judged by its staff. The points above are merely a few pointers to developing a policy that will enable all those involved to take the best decisions in relation to the many possibilities presented by the legal system where health care staff sustain criminal injuries.

REFERENCES

Ashworth, A. and Shapland, J. (1980) Psychopaths in the criminal process. *Criminal Law Review*, 628–40.
Barnett v. Chelsea and Kensington Hospital Management Committee (1969) [1969] 1 Q.B. 428.

British Psychological Society (1985) A code of conduct for psychologists. *Bulletin of The British Psychological Society*, **38**, 41–43.

Caparo Industries plc v. Dickman (1990) [1990] 2 A.C. 605.

Charlton v. Forrest Ink Printing (1980) [1980] IRLR 331.

Code for Crown Prosecutors (1992) Published as an Annex to the *Annual Report of the Crown Prosecution Service, House of Commons Paper 48*, July 1992, London.

Criminal Injuries Compensation Board (1992) *28th Annual Report for Year Ending 31 March 1992*. Cm 2122, HMSO, London.

Derrick, L. (1991) *Management Structures and Regulatory Action*. Paper given to Consultation on 'Business and Crime: Setting Standards', St George's House, Windsor Castle, September 1991, and to be published by the Faculty of Law, Sheffield University.

Doe v. Board of Commissioners of Police for Metropolitan Toronto (1989) 58 D.L.R. (4th) 396.

Ellis v. Home Office (1953) [1953] 2 All E.R. 149.

Fennell, P. (1991) Diversion of mentally disordered offenders from custody. Criminal Law Review, 333–48.

GMC (1987) *Professional Conduct and Discipline: Fitness to Practise*, General Medical Council, London.

Greer, D. (1991) *Criminal Injuries Compensation*, Sweet and Maxwell, London.

Halford v. Brookes (1991) *The Times*, 3 October 1991 [1991] 3 All E.R. 559.

Health and Safety Executive (1989) *Violence to Staff*, (ref. IND(G)69L), Health and Safety Executive, London.

Hill v. Chief Constable of West Yorkshire (1989) [1989] A.C. 53.

Hoge, S. and Gutheil, T. (1987) The prosecution of psychiatric patients for assaults on staff: a preliminary empirical study. *Hospital and Community Psychiatry*, **38**, 44–49.

Hoggett, B. (1990) *Mental Health Law*, Sweet and Maxwell, London.

Holgate v. Lancashire Mental Hospitals Board (1937) [1937] 4 All E.R. 19.

Home Office (1988) *Guidelines on Compensation in the Criminal Courts*, Home Office Circular 85/1988, London.

Home Office (1990a) *Guidelines on the Cautioning of Offenders*, Home Office Circular 59/1990, London.

Home Office (1990b) *Provision for Mentally Disordered Patients*, Home Office Circular 66/1990, London.

Home Office (1993) *Criminal Statistics: England and Wales 1991*, Cm 2134, HMSO, London.

Home Office v. Dorset Yacht Co. (1970) [1970] A.C. 1004.

Jones, M. (1990) Medical confidentiality and the public interest. *Professional Negligence*, 16–24 March.

Lane v. Holloway (1968) [1968] 1 Q.B. 379.

Mason, J. and McCall Smith, R. (1991). *Law and Medical Ethics*, Butterworths, London.

Miers, D. (1990) *Compensation for Criminal Injuries*, Butterworths, London.

Miller, R. and Maier, G. (1987) Factors affecting the decision to prosecute mental patients for criminal behavior. *Hospital and Community Psychiatry*, **38**, 50–55.

Moxon, D., Corkery, J. and Hedderman, C. (1992) *Developments in the Use of Compensation Orders in Magistrates' Courts since October 1988*, Home Office Research Study 126, HMSO, London.

Newburn, T. (1988) *The Use and Enforcement of Compensation Orders*, Home Office Research Study 102, HMSO, London.

Newburn, T. and de Peyrecave, H. (1987) Victims' attitudes to courts and compensation. *Home Office Research Bulletin*, **23**, 24–27.

P. and others v. Harrow London Borough Council (1992) *The Times*, 22 April 1992.

Poyner, B. and Warne, C. (1988) *Preventing Violence to Staff*, Health and Safety Executive. HMSO, London.

R. v. Crozier (1990) *The Independent*, 11 May 1990.

Shapland, J., Wilmore, J. and Duff, P. (1985) *Victims in the Criminal Justice System*, Gower, Aldershot.

Tarasoff v. Regents of the University of California (1974) 529 P.2d 553, 118 Cal.R 129.

West Bromwich Building Society v. Townsend (1983) [1983] IRLR 147.

W. v. Egdell (1990) [1990] Ch. 359.

W. v. Meah (1986) [1986] 1 All E.R. 935.

ACKNOWLEDGEMENTS

We wish to acknowledge the assistance given to us in the preparation of this chapter by Mr Stephen Miles of the Accident and Emergency Department at St Bartholomew's Hospital, and by Mr Phil Fennell and Mrs Vivienne Harpwood, both of Cardiff Law School. None of them has any responsibility for what is written here.

PART THREE

Prevention and management of violence at work

CHAPTER 8

The prediction of violence in a health care setting

Richard Whittington and Til Wykes

INTRODUCTION

One of the most important ways of tackling the problem of violence to health service staff is to improve our ability to predict when such violence is likely to occur. The health care professional is faced with a continuous stream of new patients or clients and staff need to know with some degree of accuracy which, if any, of these patients is likely to assault them during their period of contact. Currently such judgements are often based on clinical intuition and may be more or less accurate but there is growing evidence that more objective information could aid our predictions of violent behaviour.

PREDICTING WHEN VIOLENCE IS LIKELY TO TAKE PLACE

Several studies have attempted to estimate whether staff are able to accurately predict future violence by clients. One approach has been to interview staff after a violent incident in a psychiatric hospital and ask them whether they had anticipated or expected the violent behaviour to occur. Estimates of unpredictability (i.e. the proportion of incidents that were not predicted by staff) range from one-third to the vast majority (e.g. Cooper *et al.*, 1983; Convey, 1986). In a different setting, Breakwell and Rowett (1989) interviewed a group of residential social workers who had been assaulted and 50% reported that the incident had been completely unpredictable. The conclusion from these studies seems to be that a large number of assaults are not anticipated by staff, even though the staff may have been experienced and qualified in assessing people's behaviour.

Another, more sophisticated, approach to answering this question has been used in a group of US studies, where patients admitted to a (psychiatric) hospital were assessed on admission using a variety of measures and then the likelihood of the patient being aggressive in the 7 days following admission was estimated. This estimate was then compared with the actual occurrence of violence over the same time period. In the study by Werner *et al.* (1983a), 30 psychiatrists and psychologists based their estimates on: (i) information about the patients' mental state on admission assessed via a widely used measure of mental illness – the Brief Psychiatric Rating Scale (BPRS), and (ii) the presence or absence of violence prior to admission. Werner *et al.* (1983a) report that:

> on the whole, the judges were successful in identifying approximately two out of every five patients who would become violent (and) that on the average about one in four patients who did not become assaultive during the study period were labelled as violent.
>
> (*Werner* et al., *1983a*)

Essentially the erroneous predictions occurred because the judges used the wrong cues as indicators of violent behaviour. Of the 12 predictors thought relevant by judges (11 BPRS symptoms and the occurrence of violence prior to admission) only one, motor retardation or reduced activity/movement, was found to correlate with actual violent behaviour. Janofsky *et al.* (1988) report a similar study and again the two psychiatrists who acted as judges were relatively inaccurate in their predictions of physical assault. The psychiatrists in this study collected demographic and historical data and performed an examination of mental state. There was no correlation between predictions and actual physically assaultive behaviour but there was a significant correlation between the psychiatrists' predictions and threatening behaviour by the patients.

In contrast to these pessimistic findings, a recent study has reported more encouraging results. McNiel and Binder (1991) found that a group of nurses and psychiatrists made relatively accurate predictions about the probability of violence. The basis for their predictions was all the information collected on patients at admission but, in this study, instead of asking staff a simple yes/no prediction, they were allowed to make estimates of the probability of violence. A significant association was found between predictions by both nurses and doctors and actual violent behaviour by the patients. Ratings of nurses and doctors were significantly correlated with each other, although the prediction was somewhat stronger for the nurses. Unfortunately, after finding staff who can make relatively accurate predictions, McNiel and Binder (1991) do not give further information about the bases used for making those judgements.

In summary, the findings of these three studies are inconsistent. It is apparent that some staff who are highly trained in observing and understanding human behaviour are nevertheless relatively inaccurate at estimating the risk of aggressive behaviour by patients over a relatively short time period. Often there is no correlation between predictions and behaviour over 7 days, the majority of violent patients are not identified and one-quarter of patients are mistakenly labelled as violent. Even immediately prior to assaults, staff in the different studies had not predicted the violence in 50–97% of cases. It may be that the innovations introduced by McNiel and Binder (1991), allowing probability estimates and using nursing staff as judges, may account for the improved accuracy of predictions in their study. Whatever the explanation, there is clearly a need for further studies of this sort, especially with UK samples and preferably including nonpsychiatric patients.

One reason why the judges in the studies reported above were often inaccurate may be that they based their prediction entirely on the characteristics of the individual patient and ignored other factors that may influence the occurrence of aggressive behaviour. For instance, the mental state of the patient is obviously an important factor but there may be influences external to the patient that may also make violence more likely to occur. Psychologists have recognized for many years that situational factors are an important influence on aggressive behaviour and therefore should be included in any predictions that seek to be reasonably accurate (Archer and Browne, 1989). Baron (1977) and Geen (1990) have both reviewed studies of aggressive behaviour and discuss a wide variety of such variables. These include interpersonal factors such as frustration or attack by other people and environmental factors such as noise or crowding. Therefore, if the prediction of violence in a health care setting is to be improved, it seems necessary to include information on these other aspects of the violent situation as well as information on the violent individual.

FACTORS THAT MAY INDICATE THE LIKELIHOOD OF VIOLENCE

Since there are a wide variety of potentially relevant factors, it is convenient to attempt to categorize them in some way. A model of violence at work proposed by Poyner and Warne (1986) is particularly suitable for these purposes. Poyner and Warne were commissioned by the Health and Safety Executive (HSE) to study reports of violent incidents from a wide variety of occupational settings. The HSE initiative is part of a general governmental strategy reflecting concern about this problem, especially with regard to the NHS and social services (HSAC, 1987; DHSS, 1988). A series of case studies based on the model have also been published (Poyner and Warne, 1988).

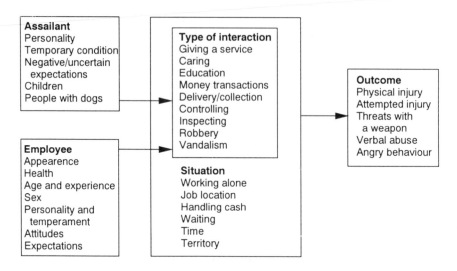

Figure 8.1 An elaborated model of violent assaults at work (from Poyner and Warne, 1986).

One of the main attractions of this model is that it seeks to be applicable to all work settings and therefore should, at least, be relevant to all the different settings in which health care professionals work, for example psychiatric hospitals, general hospitals and the community. The model is illustrated in Figure 8.1 above.

The model is relatively simple but includes a wide range of factors. Four factors in particular are seen as potentially important contributors to the occurrence of violence at work. These are aspects of: (i) the assailant; (ii) the employee; (iii) the situational context of the job, and (iv) the type of interaction that takes place between the assailant and the employee prior to the assault. It seems likely that prediction of violence in the health care setting can only begin to approach a useful level of accuracy if it is based on information about each of these contributory factors, rather than focusing narrowly on aspects of the assailant alone as occurred in the studies discussed above. Three of the four factors will now be discussed and the extent to which useful information can be derived from them for prediction will be assessed.

The assailant – who is likely to be violent?

The first element in the model is the assailant, the individual person who assaults the employee or health care professional. In most cases, this will be the patient or client for whom the staff member is providing care, although assaults by visitors and relatives of patients are by no means unknown. It was noted that the aggressive individual has been extensively studied by psychologists and is often focused upon exclusively in studies of violence in psychiatric hospitals. Many different aspects of violent individuals have been investigated including genetic inheritance and sociocultural expectations (Geen, 1990). A wide array of characteristics of violent psychiatric patients have also been studied, ranging from the experience of childhood discipline (Yesavage, 1984) to behaviour immediately prior to the assault (Aiken, 1984). Some of these factors have been found to identify violent individuals quite well while others are no more prevalent in aggressive individuals than the rest of the population and therefore are of little use for prediction.

Personality and history of violence

Firstly, Poyner and Warne (1986) propose that certain people 'react more aggressively or violently than the average' and thus may have a history of violent behaviour. They consider this propensity to aggressive behaviour as an aspect of the person's personality and there is indeed evidence that 'aggressive personalities are a reality' (Geen, 1990).

Some such personality traits that have been investigated with reference to aggressive inclinations include locus of control, Type A behaviour pattern and undercontrol/overcontrol. However, a study of patients who were aggressive in a District General Hospital psychiatric unit did not support the idea that such patients were unusual in terms of personality traits (Edwards et al., 1988). It may be that such a propensity for aggressive behaviour is as much due to social skill deficits as to these hypothesized personality traits. Furthermore, the usefulness of the concept of personality in prediction for health care professionals is extremely limited since such detailed information is rarely available to staff.

On the other hand, Poyner and Warne's (1986) suggestion that a history of violence is an effective predictor of future violent behaviour is undoubtedly true (Olweus, 1984). Also, in contrast to personality measures, information on past violent behaviour is more likely to be available in the form of records and reports (however accurate or inaccurate these may be) and therefore is more useful as a predictor. Aiken (1984), for instance, reports that all but one of the 19 patients in his study who assaulted staff had a history of previous violence.

Recent violence may be particularly useful as a guide to the risk of violence faced by staff. Many patients arriving at a hospital have been referred by other agencies who have carried out an assessment, which may include information on violent behaviour just prior to the admission, whether this is a factor in the referral or not. Most studies have indeed found that violence immediately prior to admission was predictive of violence in the early stages of an admission (e.g. McNiel *et al.*, 1988; Blomhoff *et al.*, 1990). Thus there is evidence to suggest that psychiatric patients who have been violent just before admission present a greater risk to staff than nonviolent patients.

Use of alcohol and drugs

While such concepts as 'personality' and 'social skills deficits' are relatively fixed characteristics of individuals, Poyner and Warne (1986) also propose that certain temporary conditions are influential on aggressive behaviour. Patients who are intoxicated with alcohol or drugs or, conversely, those in a state of withdrawal may present a particular risk to staff. Alcohol reduces the person's ability to make complex interpretations and increases the influence of strong situational stimuli. Illegal drugs such as marijuana, amphetamines and cocaine have been linked to violence in crimes to acquire money or the drug, although only heroin use has been linked to nonacquisitive crimes of violence such as rape. It is also possible that people in a state of withdrawal from an addictive drug (including benzodiazepines) may be more at risk of acting aggressively, if only to get access to the desired drug.

While intoxicated patients are more likely to be encountered by community staff and those in accident and emergency departments, ward staff should also be aware of the possible risks entailed by the use of some therapeutic drugs. Ochitill (1983) implicates some drugs in the causation of violence in general hospitals because of their effects on mood states. Some psychoactive drugs may have paradoxical effects on patients' behaviour including, for instance, disinhibition, increased excitation and an impaired ability to appreciate the social deviance of behaviours.

Physical and mental illness

Another temporary condition that may influence aggressive behaviour and which is obviously highly relevant to health care staff is the presence of illness in the patient. Almost by definition, the patients and clients with whom health staff interact will be suffering from some form of physical or mental illness and certain types of illness may be associated with an increased risk of aggression.

The relationship between the experience of physical illness and aggressive behaviour has very rarely been studied since violence in general hospitals has not been widely acknowledged as a significant problem. Nevertheless, physically ill patients can present a risk of assault to health care staff. In a survey of the NHS (HSAC, 1987) discussed in more detail later, 9% of staff in general hospitals reported receiving physical injury from assault by a patient over a 12-month period. The rate of assault on surgical wards was 11% and that on medical wards was 26%, the latter rate being higher than that in accident and emergency departments (20%) and equivalent to that experienced by psychiatric staff. The context and reasons for such assaults are not clear but a small US study by Ochitill (1983) may illuminate some of the factors involved.

Ochitill (1983) studied violence in the San Francisco General Hospital. Almost all violence took place in the first 10 days following admission and the frequency increased at night. It is noteworthy, in comparison, that in psychiatric settings it has been consistently found (e.g. Noble and Rodger, 1989) that violence **decreases** at night. Ochitill (1983) surmises that the reason for his findings is that the night:

> ... is a time when patients are usually less distracted from the reality of their pain, the implications of their illness and the persistent worries about other aspects of their life. The hospital wards tend to be less well staffed during these hours, reducing the availability of nurses.
>
> *(Ochitill, 1983)*

The patient's experience of pain is thus seen as an important stimulus to violent behaviour by general hospital patients. The contribution of inescapable pain to the production of violent behaviour is well known (Owens and Bagshaw, 1985). Ochitill (1983) discusses how the experience of chronic pain conditions leads to anger and hostility and reports that many incidents in his study resulted from conflicts between staff and patient over pain management.

Unlike violence in general hospitals, violence by psychiatric patients has become widely acknowledged as a significant problem. An extensive research effort has been conducted in order to identify the individual characteristics that may help predict the likelihood of violence by these patients. Not surprisingly, much of this effort has been directed at the mental illness of the patient.

When assessments of mental illness on admission are compared with the actual occurrence of aggression shortly following admission, certain relevant symptoms have been identified. First, the **overall level of psychopathology** on admission has been found to be higher in patients who subsequently become aggressive than in those who do not become aggressive (e.g. Lowenstein *et al.*, 1990). Second, there is some indication that patients presenting with psychotic features may present more risk than other patients. In particular, the admission symptoms most consistently reported as being significant predictors of subsequent violence are **conceptual disorganization** (e.g. confused, disconnected, disrupted thought processes), **hallucinatory behaviour** (e.g. perceptions without normal external stimulus correspondence) and **unusual thought content** (e.g. odd, strange or bizarre thoughts) (e.g. Janofsky *et al.*, 1988; Palmstierna *et al.*, 1989; Lowenstein *et al.*, 1990). Patients exhibiting these symptoms may be prone to aggression presumably due to their impaired ability to interpret their own and other people's behaviour appropriately. In contrast, certain symptoms have been found to be negatively associated with violent behaviour, most notably motor retardation (e.g. slowed, weakened movements or speech, reduced body tone).

While mental state on admission seems to be useful as a predictor of violence, the mental state of the inpatient seems less predictive. Krakowski *et al.* (1988) found that level of psychopathology was not significantly correlated with the frequency of violent behaviour during the admission. However, they found that social dysfunction (i.e. not participating in ward activities) was correlated with violence. Psychosis may be an important factor since Noble and Rodger (1989) found that a higher proportion of violent UK patients were hallucinated and deluded compared with nonviolent patients.

Staff should also be aware that overt hostility and suspiciousness have not always been found to be predictive of subsequent violence when these attitudes might be expected to be a useful predictor (Yesavage *et al.*, 1981). Krakowski *et al.* (1988) in fact found that hostile and suspicious behaviour was associated with lower rates of violence. This relationship between verbal and physical aggression will be explored later.

Summary

There is evidence that patients who:

- have a history of previous violence (especially if this occurred recently);
- are intoxicated;
- are in pain and/or;
- are mentally ill (especially psychotic);

present an increased risk of acting aggressively to health care staff.

The employee – who is likely to be assaulted?

A second approach to prediction is to alert those groups of staff who are most at risk of being assaulted owing to the type of patients they work with or their occupational role. In the UK, the most important source of information on violence in the NHS is the Health and Safety Commission survey (HSAC,1987), which revealed that violence is widespread across a variety of general hospital, psychiatric hospital and community settings. Several findings of this survey are worth

noting. Firstly, assaults resulting in major physical injury were relatively rare (experienced by one in 200 staff over 12 months) but assaults
resulting in minor injury were remarkably common across a wide
variety of NHS settings. No NHS specialty was exempt from either
verbal or physical aggression of some sort over a 12-month period.

Obviously the risks in certain specialties were higher than in others.
Major physical injury was most common in mental handicap,
psychiatric hospitals and accident and emergency departments. **Minor
physical injury** was sustained by more than one in 10 staff working
in geriatric, mental handicap and psychiatric settings, and the accident
and emergency department, orthopaedic, surgical and medical wards
of general hospitals. **Threats with a weapon** were made against nearly
a quarter of accident and emergency staff and one in 10 psychiatric
staff, while **verbal abuse and threats** were experienced by more than
one-third of staff in medical wards and over half of staff in accident
and emergency departments.

In staff working in the community, the HSAC (1987) survey indicates
relatively low levels of physical assault but high levels of verbal
aggression. While only about 3% of such staff had been physically
assaulted, nearly one in five had been threatened or verbally abused
in the 12 months preceding the survey. Ambulance staff appear to
be particularly at risk in the community, with 17% reporting minor
injury and 42% reporting threats in the 12 months preceding the
survey.

There is relatively little research on the context of violence to staff
in the community (although see Chapter 4). Haffke and Reid (1983)
report a study of violence in community mental health centres in the
US state of Nebraska. They supported the HSAC (1987) finding that
physical violence was relatively uncommon in this setting, with 34
incidents occurring over 2 years. The secretary or receptionist of the
centre was the target of assault in nearly one-quarter of incidents and
the police were called to respond to one-third of the incidents. Staff
pointed out the proximity of the mental health centres to local bars
with the associated risk of intoxicated clients. They were also fearful
of retribution by clients outside the workplace, for example on the
way home. Breakwell and Rowett (1989) included some field social
workers in their survey and found such staff were assaulted by a high
proportion of female clients, many of whom were mentally ill and the
assaults often took place in the client's home.

So far, prediction based on the location of work (hospital or
community) and the type of patients being cared for has been discussed. In addition, certain occupational groups may face higher risks
of assault than others regardless of the above factors. Ambulance staff
were mentioned and there is evidence that nursing staff are also
assaulted quite frequently. Student nurses, staff nurses and charge

nurses were all assaulted at least three times as often as hospital doctors in the HSAC (1987) survey and the first group suffered particularly high rates of assault (36% received physical injury, 40% were threatened or verbally abused over 12 months). Studies of violence in psychiatric settings (e.g. Noble and Rodger, 1989) demonstrate consistently that around 90% of assaults on staff are directed against nurses. This finding is not explained by the large number of nurses in the workforce compared with the number in other occupational groups (Roscoe, 1987) nor is it due to the relatively long periods nurses spend in face-to-face contact with patients (Whittington and Wykes, 1991). The most likely explanation for the increased risk of assault faced by nurses lies in the type of interaction that inevitably takes place between nurses and patients. Other research indicates that psychologists face high levels of assault. Perkins (1991) reports that over half the psychologists she surveyed had experienced physical violence at some stage in their careers and nearly one-fifth (17.7%) had been assaulted in the preceding year.

Some authors go further than examining just the workplace and occupational group of assaulted staff and suggest that there is something about certain individual members of staff that makes them more prone to be involved in violent incidents (Haller and Deluty, 1988; Lanza *et al.*, 1991). This belief is often held by staff themselves. Breakwell and Rowett (1989) found that nearly 80% of assaulted and nonassaulted social workers believed staff who were assaulted could be distinguished by certain personal characteristics such as being 'more provocative, incompetent, authoritarian and inexperienced'.

Poyner and Warne (1986) also propose that factors such as the age and sex of the employee, their appearance and other psychological attributes (e.g. mental health, personality, attitudes and expectations) may 'influence the behaviour and attitudes of the public (and) may relate to assaults'. This is a controversial claim to make since such a proposition can easily become a case of 'blaming the victim'. Furthermore, there is limited research evidence to support the claim. When researchers have studied the characteristics of assaulted and nonassaulted staff in psychiatric settings there is no consensus on whether male or female staff are assaulted more frequently (Larkin *et al.*, 1988; Carmel and Hunter, 1989; Hodgkinson *et al.*, 1985) nor is there a tendency for larger or smaller staff or younger staff to be attacked (Lanza *et al.*, 1991; Whittington, 1992). Personality traits such as hostility, neuroticism, extraversion and risk-taking also do not seem to be unusually common in assaulted staff (Edwards *et al.*, 1988; Whittington, 1992).

It seems likely, as suggested by Poyner and Warne (1986), that staff who are excessively stressed or 'burnt out' may be more at risk of being assaulted than their colleagues. Stress or mental illness in staff may impair their ability to assess adequately potentially dangerous situations and to interact skilfully in such situations (e.g. they may have a reduced ability to tolerate difficult or frustrating patients).

The type of interaction – are certain interactions dangerous?

Rather than studying the individual characteristics of assaulted staff it may be more fruitful to investigate whether certain types of interaction precede aggressive incidents. Several studies of violence in psychiatric settings support the idea that a significant proportion of incidents are preceded and therefore possibly 'triggered' by staff–patient interaction of some sort (Sheridan *et al.*, 1990; Colenda and Hamer, 1991).

Poyner and Warne (1986) place the type of interaction between staff and public at the heart of their model of violence at work but they only mention 'caring' as the relevant interaction for health care staff. This is clearly insufficient either as an explanation of why violence occurs in the health care setting or as a description of the wide variety of interactions health care professionals may have with patients. Caring takes many forms and often may be perceived as unwelcome by the patient or client. Three possible high-risk interactions in which staff may engage in order to deliver care to patients will now be discussed.

Frustration

Frustration or the 'thwarting of an ongoing, goal-directed behaviour' is an influential hypothesis for the causation of violence and many of the staff–patient conflicts in the study by Sheridan *et al.* (1990) involved frustration of the patient in some way. These frustrations included staff 'not allowing the patient to smoke (or) telling the patient to stay out of another patient's room'. Whittington and Wykes (1991) found that about one-third of assaults on staff in a UK psychiatric hospital were preceded by the victim frustrating the patient in some way. One of the most common scenarios is that in which staff in a psychiatric unit have to prevent a detained patient from leaving (Convey, 1986).

While frustration is more likely to be a problem in psychiatric settings, there may be occasions when staff in other health care roles inevitably have to frustrate their patients in some way. The example given by Ochitill (1983) of staff perceived as witholding pain relief in a general hospital could be construed in this way. Hobbs (Chapter 4) also reports the importance of being kept waiting as a factor in a large number of assaults.

Activity demand

While stopping patients doing things is one way in which they may be angered or annoyed by staff, another involves insisting that they engage in some activity when they are reluctant to do so. Sheridan *et al.* (1990) report examples of violence preceded by staff 'asking the patient to go to bed, and telling the patient to sign in'. Cooper and Medonca (1991) also found that requesting a patient to engage in some behaviour occurred before several assaults. Similarly, Aiken (1984) describes two assaults preceded by 'encouraging the patient to get out of bed'. These staff behaviours may relate to a concept of 'activity/demand' that:

> ... views physical assaultive tendencies among psychiatric patients in part as a nonverbal response made to resist or thwart another's demands. Physical assault is seen as one expression among a number of behaviors ... that communicate non-acceptance of a demand made by another (and) is understood as the consequence of a prior demand made on the striker.
>
> *(Depp, 1976)*

Thus, as with frustration, the member of staff annoys or angers the patient in order to provide 'care'. Again, such scenarios are not limited to the psychiatric settings where the above research took place. It seems likely that any sort of rehabilitation environment will involve encouraging patients who may be unwilling to be active and therefore will run some risk of aggressive behaviour.

Intrusiveness or perceived attack

A third type of interaction that may precede violence by patients might be called intrusiveness or perceived attack. In this case, the patient or client becomes aggressive because they perceive some sort of verbal or physical attack is being made upon them by staff. Actual attacks on patients by staff are few but not unknown (Martin, 1984). However, the emphasis here is on the patient's perception or 'appraisal' (Lazarus and Folkman, 1984) of the staff behaviour. Verbal attack may be perceived if staff insult, threaten or otherwise reject the patient. As mentioned above, staff experiencing high levels of stress or burnout may be particularly prone to such critical attitudes (Maslach and Jackson, 1986).

Physical intrusiveness is an even greater problem since much of the care delivered by health staff inevitably involves initiating physical contact with patients. Patients may perceive staff who simply approach them and encroach on their personal space as making some form of attack upon them and they may be particularly prone to such perceptions when distressed. Long (1984) showed that people in a high-tension situation (e.g. a dentist's waiting room) indicate a preference for greater interpersonal distance than people in low-tension situations (e.g. a television lounge). This may be particularly true for psychotic patients (Aiken, 1984; Smith and Cantrell, 1988).

In addition, some health care procedures are more likely to be perceived as an attack because they actually result in pain for the patient (e.g. giving an injection). It is clearly important therefore that patients are informed of the nature of the procedure to enable them to appraise the interaction more appropriately and that their consent is obtained where possible prior to physically intruding in this way.

Summary

Staff working in certain health care settings are more at risk of assault. However, complacency should be avoided since violence to staff occurs in every speciality of the NHS and involves staff from every occupational group. As well as being alert to these risks, staff should be aware that some of the interactions they have with patients in order to deliver care may increase the likelihood of violence occurring. Risk is likely to be increased if staff have to frustrate a patient, demand that they engage in some activity, criticize the patient or physically intrude on them.

WARNING SIGNS OF IMMINENT VIOLENCE

Many guidelines for staff working with violent patients include lists of behaviours that staff can use to predict imminent aggressive behaviour. For instance, Kronberg (1983) suggests:

> Warning signals that may be observed when 'fight' is chosen include clenched fists, walking briskly, continuous pacing, throwing items, an exaggerated response to annoyance, yelling, pressured and curt speech, quivering of the lips, rigid muscle tension, biting and scratching.
>
> (*Kronberg, 1983*)

Such guidelines are useful to direct care staff but their accuracy is often questionable. Usually, the specified behaviours have been derived from clinical observation in highly stressful circumstances and, in addition, it is possible that not all violent patients exhibit the same signs of imminent violence. Therefore, empirical data on the behavioural cues of imminent violence need to be collected in much the same way as information on the threatening behaviours by animals have been studied (Lorenz, 1966). Fortunately, a few studies have attempted to do this and these will presently be reviewed.

Firstly, it is reassuring to know that violence rarely takes place 'out of the blue', in other words without some behavioural change immediately beforehand. Only 4% of the incidents in the study by Sheridan *et al.* (1990) and less than 10% of assaults on staff in that by Aiken (1984) occurred in the absence of any observed behavioural cues. However, it is interesting that some assaults in the latter study were preceded by behavioural changes while staff still felt they had not anticipated the assault. The conclusion must be that these staff were not aware of the correct warning signs since they observed change but did not anticipate violence.

General behaviour and mental state

Sheridan *et al.* (1990) investigated the immediate precursors of violent behaviour, which led to physical restraint of a patient. Patient anxiety was very common prior to the incident (preceding 75% of incidents) with hostility (53%) and delusions (30%) less common. Hallucinations (7%) and confusion (4%) were quite rare as precursors. Lee *et al.* (1989) report that over two-thirds of the 34 patients who were violent in their study had been described as 'hyperactive, loud, verbally abusive, angry or hostile' in the notes prior to being assaultive. Other behaviour patterns (e.g. anxious, apprehensive, depressed, withdrawn, isolated, lethargic, confused, hallucinating, delusional, disorganized, bizarre behaviours) were observed prior to less than 15% of violent acts.

Verbal aggression and threats

If a patient threatens violence then they are likely to carry out the threat. Werner *et al.* (1983b) report a significant association between verbal assault (e.g. aggressive, hostile or threatening statements) by patients and physical assault over a 7-day period. Of the 38 patients, 12 (32%) who had been verbally hostile were subsequently physically aggressive in the next 7 days. Conversely, 12 of the 15 patients (80%) who were physically assaultive had preceded their assault with verbal aggression. From this we can infer that only a small group of violent patients do not give some verbal warning of impending violence. Tanke and Yesavage (1984) developed the distinction between threatening and nonthreatening violent patients a stage further by identifying significant differences in the mental states of the two groups.

The time lapse between cue behaviour and violence in both these studies was quite high, being up to 7 days in the study by Werner *et al.* (1983b) and 1–2 days in the study by Tanke and Yesavage (1984). In a UK study, Aiken (1984) interviewed staff who had been assaulted about three different aspects of patient behaviour **immediately** prior to a violent incident. Changes in one of these aspects, verbal behaviour, were highly indicative of imminent violence. 81% of assaults were preceded by a change in verbal behaviour, with nearly half preceded by loud and/or threatening behaviour.

Loud and frequent cursing preceded 51% of the incidents investigated by Sheridan *et al.* (1990) but another form of verbal behaviour, paranoid statements, preceded only about 8% of incidents. Dietz and Rada (1983) found that provocative or threatening verbal behaviour was the most common precursor of violence. However, they point out this occurred prior to few incidents and that such behaviour is so common in the forensic setting where they worked that the behaviour is of little predictive value. In another UK study, Armond (1982) reports that shouting at auditory hallucinations was a warning sign of imminent violence in an unspecified number of incidents. Finally, the assaulted social workers in Breakwell and Rowett's (1989) survey reported that 42% of assaults were immediately preceded by verbal abuse and 25% by threats.

Changes in activity and posture

Another behavioural cue that has been studied, although less frequently than verbal behaviour, is a change in the level of activity or posture of the patient prior to becoming violent. Aiken (1984) found this to be almost as common a precursor of violence as changes in verbal behaviour. In his study, 78% of assaults were preceded by a change of activity or adoption of a threatening stance. Sheridan *et al.* (1990) also found that 49% of incidents in their study were preceded by the patient 'pacing' and Lee *et al.* (1989) include 'hyperactivity' in their profile of behaviour preceding violent incidents.

It is extremely important to reiterate that some incidents in Aiken's (1984) study were preceded by the sudden cessation of activity rather than increased activity. The 'common sense' view is that all violence is preceded by increased motor activity and one of the benefits of conducting research is this demonstration that reduced activity may be as indicative of aggression as the opposite pattern.

Invasion of personal space

A further aspect investigated by Aiken (1984) is the reduction of interpersonal distance by the patient prior to being aggressive. This was found to occur much less frequently than changes in verbal behaviour or activity levels, with less than half of assaults preceded by the patient approaching less than 2 feet or one arm's length from the victim.

Summary

Aggression to health care staff rarely occurs unpredictably and 'out-of-the-blue'. Certain behaviours indicate that patients may be about to become aggressive. While some of these are well known risk factors (e.g. increased motor activity, verbal abuse) staff should be aware that any significant **change** from normal behaviour should be taken seriously. This includes sudden silence and reduced motor activity.

CONCLUSIONS

In this chapter, several factors that may help health staff to predict the likelihood of a patient they encounter becoming aggressive toward them have been reviewed. A summary of some indicators of potential violence in a health care setting is as follows:

1. The patient who is:
   (a) known to have a history of violence, especially recent violence;
   (b) intoxicated;
   (c) in pain;
   (d) mentally ill, especially if thought disordered and/or hallucinating;
   (e) verbally abusive and/or issuing threats;
   (f) speaking in a loud voice or is suddenly silent;
   (g) overactive or suddenly stops moving.
2. The health care worker who is:
   (a) working in mental handicap, psychiatric or accident and emergency settings;
   (b) a nurse or ambulance staff;
3. The type of interaction where the staff member has to:
   (a) frustrate the patient;
   (b) demand activity from the patient;
   (c) intrude on and/or touch the patient.

REFERENCES

Aiken, G.J.M. (1984) Assaults on staff in a locked ward: prediction and consequences. *Medicine, Science and the Law,* **24,** 199–207.
Archer, J. and Browne, K. (eds) (1989) *Human Aggression. Naturalistic Approaches,* Routledge, London.
Armond, A.D. (1982) Violence in the semi-secure ward of a psychiatric hospital. *Medicine, Science and the Law,* **22,** 203–209.
Baron, R. (1977) *Human Aggression,* Plenum Press, New York.

Blomhoff, S., Seim, S. and Friis, S. (1990) Can prediction of violence among psychiatric inpatients be improved? *Hospital and Community Psychiatry*, **41**, 771–75.

Breakwell, G.M. and Rowett, C. (1989). Violence and social work, in *Human Aggression. Naturalistic Approaches*, (eds J. Archer and K. Browne), Routledge, London.

Carmel, H. and Hunter, M. (1989) Staff injuries from inpatient violence. *Hospital and Community Psychiatry*, **40**, 41–46.

Colenda, C.C. and Hamer, R.M. (1991) Antecedents and interventions for aggressive behavior of patients in a geriopsychiatric state hospital. *Hospital and Community Psychiatry*, **42**, 287–92.

Convey, J. (1986). A record of violence. *Nursing Times*, **82**(46), 36–38.

Cooper, A.J. and Medonca, J.D. (1991) A prospective study of patient assault on nurses in a provincial psychiatric hospital in Canada. *Acta Psychiatrica Scandinavica*, **84**, 163–66.

Cooper, S.J., Browne, F.W.A., McClean, K.J. (1983) Aggressive behaviour in a psychiatric observation ward. *Acta Psychiatrica Scandinavica*, **68**, 386–93.

Depp, F.C. (1976) Violent behavior patterns on psychiatric wards. *Aggressive Behavior*, **2**, 295–306.

DHSS (1988) *Violence to Staff. Report of the DHSS Advisory Committee on Violence to Staff*, HMSO, London.

Dietz, P.E. and Rada, R.T. (1983) Battery incidents and batterers in a maximum security hospital. *Archives of General Psychiatry*, **39**, 31–34.

Edwards, J.G., Jones, D., Reid, W.H. *et al.* (1988) Physical assaults in a psychiatric unit in a general hospital. *American Journal of Psychiatry*, **145**, 1568–71.

Geen, R.G. (1990) *Human Aggression*. Open University Press, Milton Keynes.

Haffke, E.A. and Reid, W.H. (1983) Violence against mental health personnel in Nebraska, in *Violence Within Psychiatric Facilities*, (eds J.R. Lion and W.H. Reid), Grune and Stratton, New York, pp. 91–102.

Haller, R.M. and Deluty, R.H. (1988) Assaults on staff by psychiatric inpatients. A critical review. *British Journal of Psychiatry*, **152**, 174–79.

Hodgkinson, P.E., McIvor, L. and Phillips, M. (1985) Patient assaults on staff in a psychiatric hospital: a 2-year retrospective study. *Medicine, Science and the Law*, **25**, 288–94.

HSAC (1987) *Violence to Staff in the Health Services*, HMSO, London.

Janofsky, J.S., Spears, S. and Neubauer, D.N. (1988) Psychiatrists' accuracy in predicting violent behaviour on an inpatient unit. *Hospital and Community Psychiatry*, **39**, 1090–1094.

Krakowski, M., Jaeger, J. and Volavka, J. (1988) Violence and psychopathology: a longitudinal study. *Comprehensive Psychiatry*, **29**, 174–81.

Kronberg, M.E. (1983) Nursing intervention in the management of the assaultive patient, in *Assaults within Psychiatric Facilities*, (eds J.R. Lion and W.H. Reid), Grune and Stratton, New York, pp. 225–40.

Lanza, M.L., Kayne, H.L., Hicks, C. *et al.* (1991) Nursing staff characteristics related to patient assault. *Issues in Mental Health Nursing*, **12**, 253–65.

Larkin, E., Murtagh, S. and Jones, S. (1988). A preliminary study of violent incidents in a Special Hospital (Rampton). *British Journal of Psychiatry*, **153**, 226–31.

Lazarus, R. and Folkman, S. (1984) *Stress, Appraisal and Coping*, Springer, New York.

Lee, H.K., Villar, O., Juthani, N. *et al.* (1989) Characteristics and behavior of patients involved in psychiatric ward incidents. *Hospital and Community Psychiatry*, **40**, 1295–97.

Long, G.T. (1984) Psychological tension and closeness to others: stress and interpersonal distance preference. *Journal of Psychology*, **117**, 143–46.

Lorenz, K. (1966) *On Aggression*, Methuen, London.

Lowenstein, M., Binder, R.L. and McNiel, D.E. (1990) The relationship between admission symptoms and hospital assaults. *Hospital and Community Psychiatry*, **41**, 311–13.

Martin, J.P. (1984) *Hospitals in Trouble*, Blackwell, London.

Maslach, C. and Jackson, S.E. (1986) *Maslach Burnout Inventory Manual*, 2nd edn, Consulting Psychologists Press, Palo Alto, California.

McNiel, D.E. and Binder, R.L. (1991) Clinical assessment of the risk of violence amongst psychiatric inpatients. *American Journal of Psychiatry*, **148**, 1317–21.

McNiel, D.E., Binder, R.L. and Greenfield, T.K. (1988) Predictors of violence in civilly committed acute psychiatric patients. *American Journal of Psychiatry*, **145**, 965–70.

Noble, P. and Rodger, S. (1989) Violence by psychiatric in-patients. *British Journal of Psychiatry*, **155**, 384–90.

Ochitill, H.N. (1983) Violence in a general hospital, in *Violence Within Psychiatric Facilities*, (eds J.R. Lion and W.H. Reid), Grune and Stratton, New York, pp. 103–18.

Olweus, D. (1984) Development of stable aggressive reaction patterns in males, in *Advances in the Study of Aggression, Vol. 1*, (eds R.J. Blanchard and D.C. Blanchard), Academic Press, London.

Owens, R.G. and Bagshaw, M. (1985) First steps in the functional analysis of aggression, *Current Issues in Clinical Psychology*, vol. 1 (ed. E. Karas), Gower, Aldershot.

Palmstierna, T., Lassenius, R. and Wistedt, B. (1989) Evaluation of the Brief Psychopathological Rating Scale in relation to aggressive behaviour by acute involuntarily admitted patients. *Acta Psychiatrica Scandinavica*, **79**, 313–16.

Perkins, R. (1991). *Clinical Psychologist's Experience of Violence at Work*. Paper presented at the Annual Conference of the British Psychological Society, Bournemouth, April 1991.

Poyner, B. and Warne, C. (1986) *Violence to Staff: A Basis for Assessment and Prevention*, HMSO, London.

Poyner, B. and Warne, C. (1988) *Preventing Violence to Staff*, HMSO, London.

Roscoe, J. (1987) *Survey on the Incidence and Nature of Violence Occurring in the Joint Hospitals*. Report to the Working Party on Violence, Bethlem Royal and Maudsley Hospitals Special Health Authority.

Sheridan, M., Henrion, R., Robinson, L. *et al.* (1990) Precipitants of violence in a psychiatric inpatient setting. *Hospital and Community Psychiatry*, **41**, 776–80.

Smith, B.J. and Cantrell, P.J. (1988). Distance in nurse–patient encounters. *Journal of Psychosocial Nursing and Mental Health Services*, **26**(2), 22–26.

Tanke, E.D. and Yesavage, J.A. (1984) Characteristics of assaultive patients who do and do not provide visible cues of potential violence. *American Journal of Psychiatry*, **142**, 1409–13.

Werner, P.D., Rose, T.L. and Yesavage, J.A. (1983a) Reliability, accuracy and decision-making strategy in clinical predictions of imminent dangerousness. *Journal of Consulting and Clinical Psychology*, **51**, 815–25.

Werner, P.D., Yesavage, J.A., Becker, J.M.T. *et al.* (1983b) Hostile words and assaultive behaviour on an acute inpatient psychiatric unit. *Journal of Nervous and Mental Disease*, **171**, 385–87.

Whittington, R. (1992) *Assaults on Nurses by Patients in Psychiatric Hospitals*. Unpublished PhD thesis, Department of Psychology, Institute of Psychiatry, University of London.

Whittington, R. and Wykes, T. (1991) *Psychiatric Nurses' Experience of Violence at Work*. Paper presented at the Annual Conference of the British Psychological Society, Bournemouth, April 1991.

Whittington, R. and Wykes, T. (1992) *Violence to Nurses: Do Interaction Rates Explain Why Some Grades of Nurses are More at Risk of Assault than Others?* Paper presented at the Advances in Nursing Practice and Research Conference, Institute of Psychiatry, London, May 1992.

Yesavage, J.A. (1984) Correlates of dangerous behaviour by schizophrenics in hospital. *Journal of Psychiatric Research*, **18**, 225–31.

Yesavage, J.A., Werner, P.D., Becker, J. *et al.* (1981) Inpatient evaluation of aggression in psychiatric patients. *Journal of Nervous and Mental Disease*, **169**, 299–302.

CHAPTER 9

The pharmacological management of aggressive behaviour

Lyn Pilowsky

INTRODUCTION

The violent or agitated patient situation demands immediate co-ordinated management. Violent patients pose a risk to themselves and others and medical and nursing staff have a mandate to act swiftly to bring the situation to a close before damage results. Pharmacological methods of managing violence are part of the total evaluation of the patient and complement other therapeutic tools, such as behavioural and psychosocial interventions. This chapter will concern itself solely with the drug management of violence, in particular, emergency sedation. This procedure (giving psychotropic medication) to control behavioural disturbance is one of the commonest types of emergency medication and will be referred to here as rapid tranquillization (RT; Dubin, 1988). This is to distinguish it from rapid neuroleptization, in which large doses of antipsychotics are given intravenously or intra-muscularly in an effort to rapidly curtail acute psychotic symptoms.

Ideally, RT should be titrated against the patient's response. It is reversible and safe in overdosage with a large therapeutic window. In this chapter, RT will be evaluated according to choice of drug, dose and mode of delivery.

THE EPIDEMIOLOGY AND PREDICTION OF VIOLENCE – WHICH PATIENT WILL NEED RT?

The risk of violence has been underestimated in the mentally ill (Mullen, 1988). In a survey of mentally abnormal offenders, Hafner and Boker (1982) found that schizophrenic patients were twice as much at risk of offending than other groups. The reason this is not highlighted is perhaps because many such offences do not result in criminal charges or prosecution of the offender. Within a hospital setting, violent incidents are often underreported (Haller and Deluty, 1988). The Maudsley violent incident register recorded a 3–4 fold increase in assaults from 1982 to 1987 (Noble and Rodger, 1989). In a 5-month period in the same hospital, 1217 incidents were recorded, most involving actual assaults on staff. RT was applied in 8% of cases (Pilowsky *et al.*, 1992). Tardiff and Sweillam (1980) reported on over 9000 admissions to a state mental hospital and found 21% of the patients had had trouble with violent or self-destructive behaviour and 8% had assaulted others prior to admission. Another large series (Craig, 1982), found 11% of patients had acts of violence associated with their admission. Risk factors for overt aggression and assaultiveness include verbal threats of violence before admission, and a history of actual assaults (McNiel and Binder, 1989). Much inpatient violence occurs during the active phase of psychosis early in an admission and is associated with low serum levels of neuroleptics (Yesavage, 1982). On a semi-secure forensic unit, McLaren *et al.* (1990) identified a subgroup of repeatedly violent patients not amenable to treatment with oral 'as needed' medication requiring long-term management of aggression. Sheard (1988) has reviewed this area comprehensively.

Nursing staff bear the brunt of violent attacks (Chapter 2). One study found 16/100 nurses assaulted over a year compared with 1.9/100 non-nursing staff (Carmel and Hunter, 1989). Many of the assaults were incurred during physical restraint, thus reinforcing the need for RT. Patients with a diagnosis of schizophrenia and other functional disorders (e.g. mania), are associated with violence (Tardiff and Sweillam, 1980; Madden *et al.*, 1976; McNiel and Binder, 1989; Pearson *et al.*, 1986; Barber *et al.*, 1988; Coldwell and Naismith, 1989; Fottrell, 1980). Early recognition of potentially aggressive patients may prevent violence and enhance containment if violence is imminent. One such sign is an increase in verbal and motor activity found by Aiken (1984) in a study of predictors of violence in a locked psychiatric ward.

DIAGNOSIS AND RAPID TRANQUILLIZATION

Often, nursing and medical staff believe that treatment with RT should not take place until the diagnosis is clarified. While acknowledging that differential diagnosis is crucial, this should not delay treatment in a dangerous situation. If the patient is suffering from a serious organic disorder, their violence will only worsen their physical state and impede thorough clinical and laboratory evaluation. Other illnesses associated with violence are shown in Table 9.1. This is not an exhaustive list and it must be borne in mind that any toxic or delirious state can present as violent and so staff, especially on medical or surgical wards, should be alert to this possibility (Jacobs, 1983).

Table 9.1 Psychiatric disorders associated with violence

Organic syndromes	Functional disorders
Acute brain syndrome (e.g. delirium – postsurgical, delirium tremens, diabetic stupor etc.)	Schizophrenia
Chronic brain syndrome (e.g. dementia)	Mania
Specific syndromes (e.g. episodic dyscontrol, frontal/temporal and limbic epilepsy)	Drug or alcohol abuse

Although a full history and examination may not be feasible until the situation is contained, it should be possible to glean crucial medical information from staff on the scene; for example, if there is a history of epilepsy or diabetes and the patient's current medication. The patient may exhibit obvious focal neurological signs or have clouding of consciousness. Patients who have a deterioration in their ability to communicate (i.e. who have dementia or mental impairment) may also be prone to violent behaviour.

WHEN TO APPLY RT – TARGETING SYMPTOMS

The sensible application of RT involves a systematic approach to situations or behaviours that merit drug treatment. It is not easy to maintain clinical objectivity in the face of perceived or actual threat. A stepwise plan ensures that the treatment matches the situation and prevents potentially dangerous under- or over-reactions. A plan of management is given in Table 9.2.

The approach set out in Table 9.2 is intended as a guide only. Patient assessment is an individually tailored exercise. For example, a verbally threatening patient with no history of violence who appears relaxed may only need oral medication and distraction. An aggressive patient with a known history of violence who has been physically violent but is currently relaxed will probably need RT. Nonpharmacological

Table 9.2 Guidelines for management of violence

Level of aggressive behaviour	Response	Team
Potentially violent		
Tense/restless (e.g. pacing around, glaring or staring suspiciously), past history of violence, young, male, psychotic, verbal threats, confrontation taking place	Try non-drug methods e.g. talking down/ distraction, seclusion, segregation, offer oral medication, hold injectable medication ready, plan physical restraint	One to two nurses in the room/outside the door, doctor present
Overt aggression		
Increase in motor activity, raised voice, increase in verbal threats and more directed, beginning to attack property (e.g. slamming doors or throwing cups)	May still try non-drug methods but move swiftly to physical restraint and RT if behaviour not controlled or escalating – have time limit for improvement	Three to four nurses ready to start restraint, doctor present
Actual aggression	Physical restraint and RT	Four to six nurses control and restraint, doctor present
Violence directed at people or property, requiring immediate physical restraint		

methods of behavioural control will not be discussed here but clearly physical restraint is often required in order to administer RT (Chapter 10). It is vital for patient and staff that the restraint technique be practised, competent and safe. Jacobs (1983) has outlined a routine protocol but most institutions have their own methods.

THE LAW AND RAPID TRANQUILLIZATION

Without going into the legalities of giving RT in depth, legal provision to treat against the patient's wishes in the UK is given by common law if staff believe the patient is suffering from a mental illness (organic or functional) and is an immediate danger either to themselves or others. It must also be clear that the emergency treatment will prevent serious injury to people or property. Sections 2 and 3 of the Mental Health Act 1983 also provide for cover for involuntary routine or emergency treatment. There are very few empirical data on the use of RT and most are from studies of psychiatric care. Most psychiatric patients are usually given RT while they are subject to a section of

Table 9.3 Studies evaluating drugs in the management of aggressive behaviour

Study	Drug(s)	Dose and Route	Outcome	Comments
Clinton et al. (1987)	Haloperidol	IM/IV/Oral average dose 8 mg	83% – disturbance controlled within 30 min	Open trial in an accident and emergency department 136 patients included
Resnick et al. (1984)	Haloperidol v. droperidol	IM dose 5 mg	Droperidol better than haloperidol	Double blind study 27 patients psychotic agitation
Granacher et al. (1979)	Droperidol	IM dose 6.6 mg	22 out of 24 patients responded	Open trial, patients with psychotic agitation
Donlon et al. (1979)	Haloperidol	IM dose 22 mg	Good response, high degree of safety	Open trial to assess cardio-vascular safety in a cardiac intensive care unit
Lerner et al. (1979)	Haloperidol v. diazepam	IV haloperidol 35 mg diazepam 35 mg	No difference between treatments	Single-blind trial in psychotic patients
Freinhar et al. (1986)	Clonazepam	Oral up to 3 mg/day	Effective	Case report of three patients
Chakrabarti (1983)	Haloperidol and diazepam	IV haloperidol 10 mg Diazepam 20 mg single dose	Effective sedation	Abstract, up to 60 psychotic patients, open trial
Tesar et al. (1985)	Haloperidol	IV dose up to 100 mg/day	Effective sedation	Open trial, no cardiac side-effects, used in cardiac patients
Anderson et al. (1975)	Haloperidol	IM 10–45 mg	Complete remission in 11/24 patients	Open trial, 24 psychotic patients, wide variation in dose requirement
Tuason (1986)	Loxapine v. haloperidol	IM loxapine mean dose 83 mg Haloperidol mean dose 25 mg	Loxapine same effect as haloperidol	Double-blind study in paranoid schizophrenic patients (n=54) over 24–72 h
Neff et al. (1972)	Droperidol	IM dose 5–10 mg	76% of patients responded within 30 min	Open trial, 32 patients, functional and organic psychosis
Rapp (1987)	Haloperidol and chlorpromazine	IM haloperidol 5–20 mg Chlorpromazine 25–100 mg	No information	Small descriptive survey

the Mental Health Act 1983. In one survey of emergency RT, 88% of patients were on a section of the Mental Health Act 1983 at the time of injection (Pilowsky *et al.*, 1992). Further detailed evidence of the use of RT in medical settings needs to be collected.

CHOICE OF DRUG

Examples of studies evaluating drugs in the management of aggressive behaviour are given in Table 9.3.

Antipsychotics

There have been many open studies of the use of antipsychotics to control behavioural disturbance (Neff *et al.*, 1972; Lerner *et al.*, 1979; Resnick and Burton, 1984; Tuason, 1986). In general, these drugs should be used only where sedatives alone are contraindicated (e.g. in respiratory compromise) or if the clinician wishes to give a loading dose of antipsychotic to supplement or commence definitive treatment of a psychotic illness. The major limiting factors in the use of these drugs are their safety and side-effects relative to each other, as well as flexibility in drug delivery. The most investigated and safest antipsychotics for emergencies are haloperidol and droperidol (Ellison *et al.*, 1989; Dubin, 1988, Ayd, 1978, 1980; Clinton *et al.*, 1987; Granacher and Ruth, 1979). Both haloperidol and droperidol have a low incidence of side-effects (Dubin, 1988). The cardiorespiratory safety of haloperidol is well established, even in intensive care settings (Tesar *et al.*, 1985).

Other antipsychotics, including loxapine, molindone and thioridazine, are not more efficacious than haloperidol (Goldberg *et al.*, 1989). In the elderly, promazine, a weak antipsychotic with sedative activity, has been recommended for use but there is no hard evidence to support this claim. Chlorpromazine, once the standby for treating psychotic agitation, may cause hypotension and cannot be given safely intravenously, thus limiting its flexibility.

The effectiveness of haloperidol was tested in a study of 136 patients with a variety of diagnoses (the majority suffering from alcohol intoxication or psychosis) attending a general hospital casualty. Disruptive behaviour was alleviated within 30 min in 83% of cases. One patient became seriously hypotensive but was already critically ill (Clinton *et al.*, 1987). Patients received the drug intramuscularly at a mean dose of 8 mg haloperidol (Clinton *et al.*, 1987). Although droperidol may cause transient hypotension (Ayd, 1980), this is seldom a problem in practice. It is rapidly metabolized and so is often preferred in emergencies.

Up to one-third of patients given antipsychotics will develop extrapyramidal reactions. The most serious of these, in terms of subjective distress to the patient, are acute dystonias and oculogyric crises. It may therefore be sensible to give an antiparkinsonian drug, such as procyclidine, prophylactically. Antiparkinsonian drugs are especially indicated in patients who are most prone to such reactions. These are those patients who are young, male, who have a previous history of extrapyramidal reactions, or patients with Parkinson's disease and those for whom a dystonic reaction would be dangerous such as patients in spinal traction (Goldberg *et al.*, 1989).

Several studies support the use of antipsychotics in medically delirious patients where oversedation is not desirable (Moore, 1977; Fauman, 1978; Nadelson, 1976; Blachly and Starr, 1966).

Benzodiazepines

Benzodiazepines are often used in psychiatric emergencies because of their low toxicity. They reduce the need for high doses of antipsychotics, which have been demonstrated as unnecessary and possibly toxic in the treatment of psychosis (Van Putten *et al.*, 1990). They are also useful in patients where antipsychotics are relatively contraindicated, for example those patients who are prone to seizures, or who have had idiosyncratic reactions previously. Benzodiazepines have been applied effectively to drug-induced agitation, early psychotic relapse and combined with lithium in mania (Modell *et al.*, 1985; Lerner *et al.*, 1979). The drugs most often used for emergencies are lorazepam and diazepam.

Lorazepam is a short-acting benzodiazepine with a half-life of 12–14 h. It is not eliminated by hepatic oxidation and has no active metabolites. It may be of use in patients with liver impairment or those on medications where drug interactions could be expected. Diazepam has many metabolites and a long half-life. Thus there is a rapid onset of action with a slow offset. It accumulates when given frequently and has a gradual withdrawal phase. This is important to bear in mind as large bolus doses given too quickly may cause respiratory arrest, and it should be avoided in the physically ill or delirious patient. However, the slow offset of action may be advantageous in drug or alcohol withdrawal.

Clonazepam is a benzodiazepine that has been used in the maintenance treatment of epilepsy. Recent reports have suggested it may be helpful in treating uncontrollable agitation not responsive to conventional medication at usual doses (Freinhar and Alvarez, 1986); however, it has yet to be evaluated fully for this purpose.

Paradoxical aggression has been reported following benzodiazepine use. However, a review (Dietch and Jennings, 1988) found that the incidence of irritability and aggression was less than 1%, suggesting that this phenomenon is probably a nonspecific effect. All benzodiazepines may produce confusion, ataxia and oversedation in the elderly and are best avoided. In psychosis, prescriptions should be monitored closely and benzodiazepines should not be given as maintenance therapy once the acute phase is over as dependence may develop (Salzman, 1988). Fast withdrawal of benzodiazepines may precipitate violent reactions and therefore needs to be performed carefully and monitored.

Antipsychotics and benzodiazepines

Dubin (1988) has suggested that these drugs can act synergistically when administered together to control violence. Thus the amount of both required is reduced while still resulting in a controlled patient. Pilowsky *et al.* (1992) surveyed the use of RT in 102 incidents involving 60 patients in a general psychiatric hospital and found that overt aggression scores (as defined by a 10-point overt aggression scale) declined more rapidly when antipsychotics and sedatives were used together rather than sedatives alone. Staff expressed greatest satisfaction with the outcome of the violent patient episode when the combination was used. Others have reported that combined haloperidol and lorazepam is both safe and useful in treating violent delirium associated with serious physical illness, such as end-stage cancer (Adams, 1988), and in managing disruptive patients effectively on an open general ward (Chakrabarti, 1983). The argument against combined drug treatment is that it may confuse therapies and result in accidental overdose of medication. In the survey by Pilowsky *et al.* (1992), only one patient became confused after a combination of 40 mg haloperidol, 2.5 mg lorazepam and 10 mg diazepam intravenously. In another patient, mild hypotension occurred after 5 mg diazepam and 100 mg chlorpromazine syrup were given. It would seem sensible to use monotherapy (a sedative) to control violence in the first instance, resorting to combination treatment only in persistently violent patients, or those patients who will transfer from emergency antipsychotics to maintenance therapy.

WHAT IS THE CORRECT DOSAGE IN EMERGENCIES?

There is a wide variation in response to medication, which depends on pharmacokinetic factors, for instance patient size or tolerance to the drug and, as yet undetermined, pharmacodynamic factors. Few surveys have examined dosages used in actual practice. Clinton *et al.*

(1987) found the mean dose of haloperidol used in 136 casualty patients was 8 mg. In the survey by Pilowsky *et al.* (1992) psychiatric patients were found to receive much higher doses; mean doses of commonly used drugs were: diazepam 27 mg (range 10–80 mg), haloperidol 22 mg (range 10–60 mg), droperidol 14 mg (range 10–20 mg) and chlorpromazine 162 mg (range 50–400 mg). One adverse reaction in this survey was directly attributable to overdosage (60 mg diazepam and 80 mg haloperidol as a single dose over 10 min). To minimize the danger of overdose in emergencies (which cannot be underestimated), staff should have a pre-arranged routine. An example of this would be to draw up 20 mg of diazepam and/or haloperidol in separate syringes. These may then be given in 5 mg boluses intravenously or intramuscularly every 15 min **carefully titrating dose to response**. Suggested regimens for treatment are published in the British National Formulary (1991), but are often inadequate when dealing with highly disturbed psychiatrically ill patients. They are currently under review.

ROUTE OF ADMINISTRATION

Oral medication, especially in liquid form, is desirable whenever possible. If the patient refuses oral medication or cannot take oral drugs they may be given intramuscularly or intravenously.

The bioavailability of haloperidol is increased by intramuscular compared with oral administration (Schafer *et al.*, 1982), but there have not been any prospective studies to compare the intramuscular with the intravenous route. Pilowsky *et al.* (1992) found the intravenous route produced a more rapid decline in aggression than the intramuscular route. Others who support the intravenous route point to its safety and speed of onset (Ayd, 1978; Resnick and Burton, 1984). A further advantage is that established venous access permits greater flexibility in titrating dose and response; however, this route is not available to nursing staff.

Both droperidol and lorazepam may be given intramuscularly. Diazepam should not be given into the muscle as it is absorbed unpredictably and variably (Freinhar and Alvarez, 1986). Droperidol has been shown to have almost as rapid an action given intramuscularly as intravenously, working within 5–20 min. In the treatment of manic agitation, lorazepam was shown to have greatest effect on agitation in 2 h given orally, 1 h given intramuscularly and 5–10 min given intravenously (Modell *et al.*, 1985).

In general, it would be sensible to offer oral medication if indicated, holding injectable medication to use swiftly if necessary. The speed of onset of intravenous medication suggests that it would be safer to use in emergencies, but this may not always be practical. Where possible, doctors should be present at behavioural emergencies to supervise drug management and give intravenous RT if necessary. Once immediate control of symptoms has been brought about, oral medication can be reintroduced.

AFTERCARE

The care of violent patients does not stop once the immediate danger to themselves or others is over. The sedated patient should be observed continuously with regular measurement of vital signs for at least 1 h following RT (first because cardiorespiratory depression or idio-syncratic reactions may occur after sedation and, second, because the drug effect may wear off more quickly than expected and dangerous behaviour re-emerge). Subsequent observations depend on the patient's underlying condition and their rate of recovery. The medically ill patient will require appropriate examination, investigation and treatment. Even after minor incidents, all staff should review the management of the patient and the situation. Considerable practical and psychological support may be required for staff injured or threatened during violent incidents (Chapter 5, 7 and 11). The psychiatric ward is a community so the effects of the incident on other patients should be taken into account and discussed openly at community meetings.

RT AND COMMUNITY CARE

Psychological strategies and maintenance drug therapy will need to be combined in order to manage the potentially aggressive patient in the community. One of the most important causes of aggression is psychotic relapse, so regular assessment of the mental state, with particular attention to insight and willingness to comply with antipsychotic medication, is mandatory. Clearly, injectable depot antipsychotic medication minimizes the risk of noncompliance and provides a regular setting in which monitoring can take place. There are no specific antiaggressive drug treatments available currently, although lithium or carbamazepine have been recommended for management of chronic aggression (Sheard, 1988). The new, atypical, antipsychotic clozapine is extremely effective in 30% of patients resistant to classical antipsychotics (Kane *et al.*, 1988), and may be especially helpful in those patients whose persistent psychosis is associated with behavioural disturbance. At present, it may only be prescribed by licensed psychiatrists and if routine weekly full blood counts are performed, because of the risk of agranulocytosis.

The general practitioner (GP) should attempt to identify any potentially treatable causes of aggression, for example, physical illness or drug side-effects, in particular akithisia (Crowner *et al.*, 1990). Simple psychological measures may be applied in the community. Some examples will be mentioned briefly here. Lay carers and the patient can be trained to recognize 'early warning signs' and act to defuse problems before they get out of hand. This is achieved by using neutral and tactful communication and pre-arranged limit setting, which is firmly adhered to (e.g. a 'cooling off' room where patients can retreat until they feel calmer). The carers often require considerable emotional and practical support from health professionals. The aggressive patient's demands can be acknowledged but only discussed at length when they are more settled. The carers should be positively encouraged to call for help if a dangerous situation develops. A register of potentially dangerous patients will enable the GP (and especially locums) to attend prepared, with the necessary police, psychiatric, and social work back-up.

If emergency sedation is required RT can be applied but it must be easy to deliver and safe with minimal medical supervision, for example, lorazepam 1–3 mg, or droperidol 10–20 mg intramuscularly (IM). Without suitable resuscitation equipment to hand, intravenous sedation is unwise. As already mentioned, it is never appropriate to give diazepam IM, and chlorpromazine IM is relatively contraindicated, especially if the diagnosis is unclear. The stepwise approach outlined in Table 9.2 applies equally in the community, where it may be possible to 'catch' behavioural disturbance early. Talking down may be accomplished with a calm, experienced professional, particularly if they are known and trusted by the patient. Only a doctor can apply RT against the patient's wishes, if the behaviour presents a grave risk to the patient or others.

SUMMARY

The aggressive patient will need calming. In conjunction with other methods of treatment, RT is often justified. The drug, dosage and mode of delivery are frequently chosen rapidly, in the heat of the moment. If the doctor or nurse has a clear plan of management this will prevent over- or undertreatment of the patient, both equally dangerous. It is hoped that this chapter has mapped out safe guidelines with clear rationales for emergency treatment. The following principles apply generally:

1. Risk assessment and violence prevention take priority over diagnostic evaluation, except in cases where diagnosis crucially affects immediate choice of drug and dosage (e.g. respiratory compromise).

2. The main aim of RT is control of aggressive **behaviour**, not its underlying cause; thus a sedative drug is indicated, should be administered slowly and titrated against improvement in **specific behavioural symptoms** – the ideal is to achieve a lightly sedated, co-operative patient, allowing comprehensive evaluation and treatment.

3. The drugs of choice are benzodiazepines; either lorazepam (may be given intramuscularly or intravenously; dose: 1–3 mg) or diazepam (may only be given intravenously; dose: 10–20 mg). If there is any question of respiratory insufficiency, haloperidol or droperidol are indicated (may be given intramuscularly or intravenously; dose: 10–20 mg).

RT is a last-resort treatment but one that should be administered compassionately, using the lowest possible dose to achieve the desired effect.

REFERENCES

Adams, F. (1988) Emergency Intravenous Sedation of the Delirious Medically Ill Patient, *J. Clin. Psychiatr.*, **49**(suppl.), 22–7.

Aiken, G.J.M. (1984) Assaults on staff on a locked ward: Prediction and consequences, *Med. Sci. Law*, **24**, 199–207.

Anderson, W.H., Kuehnle, J.C. and Catanzano, D.M. (1975) Rapid treatment of acute psychosis. *Am. J. Psychiatr.*, **133**, 1076–8.

Ayd, F.J. (1978) Intravenous haloperidol therapy. *Int. Drug Ther. Newsletter*, **13**.

Ayd, F.J. (1980) Parenteral (IM/IV) droperidol for acutely disturbed behaviour in psychotic and nonpsychotic individuals. *Int. Drug Ther. Newsletter*, **15**.

Barber, J.W. *et al.* (1988) Clinical and demographic characteristics of 15 patients with repetitively assaultive behaviour. *Psychiatric Quarterly*, **59**, 213–24.

Blachly, P.H. and Starr, A. (1966) Treatment of delirium with phenothiazine drugs following open heart surgery. *Dis. Nerv. Syst.*, **27**, 107–10.

British National Formulary (1991) *British National Formulary, Number 21*, The British Medical Association and The Pharmaceutical Press, London.

Carmel, H. and Hunter, M. (1989) Staff Injuries From Inpatient Violence, *Hosp. Comm. Psychiatr.*, **40**, 41–6.

Chakrabarti, G.N. (1983) Rapid Relief of Psychotic States by Intravenous Administration of Haloperidol Followed by Intravenous Diazepam, Proceedings of the VIIth World Congress Psychiatr. Vienna (Abstr.), 573.

Clinton, J.E., Sterner, S., Stelmacher, Z. *et al.* (1987) Haloperidol for sedation of disruptive emergency patients, *Ann. Emergency Med.*, **16**, 319–22.

Coldwell, J. and Naismith, L. (1989) Violent incidents in special care wards in a special hospital, *Med. Sci. Law*, **29**, 116–23.

Craig, T.J. (1982) An epidemiological study of problems associated with violence among psychiatric inpatients, *Am. J. Psychiatr.*, **139**, 1262–66.

Crowner, M.L., Doyon, R., Convit, A. *et al.* (1990) Akithisia and violence. *Psychopharm. Bull.*, **26**, 115–17.

Dietch, J.T. and Jennings, R.K. (1988) Aggressive dyscontrol in patients treated with benzodiazepines, *J. Clin. Psychiatr.*, **49**, 184–88.

Donlon, P.T., Hopkin, J. and Tupin, J.P. (1979) Overview: efficacy and safety of the rapid neuroleptization method with injectable haloperidol. *American Journal of Psychiatry*, **136**, 273–8.

Dubin, W.R. (1988) Rapid tranquillization: Antipsychotics or benzodiazepines? *Journal of Clinical Psychiatry*, **49** (Suppl. 12), 5–12.

Ellison, J., Hughes, D. and Kimberly, A.W. (1989) An emergency psychiatry update. *Hosp. Comm. Psychiatr.*, **40**, 250–60.

Fauman, M.A. (1978) Treatment of the agitated patient with an organic brain disorder. *JAMA*, **240**, 380.

Fottrell, E. (1980) A study of violent behaviour among patients in psychiatric hospitals. *Brit. J. Psychiatr.*, **136**, 216–21.

Freinhar, J.P. and Alvarez, W.A. (1986) Clonazepam treatment of organic brain syndromes in three elderly patients, *J. Clin. Psychiatr.*, **47**, 525–26.

Goldberg, R.J., Dubin, W.R. and Fogel, B.S. (1989) Review: Behavioural emergencies, assessment and psychopharmacologic management, *Clin. Neuropharmacol.*, **12**, 233–48.

Granacher, R.P. and Ruth, D.D. (1979) Droperidol in acute agitation, *Curr. Ther. Res.* **25**, 361–65.

Hafner, H. and Boker, W. (1982) *Crimes of Violence by Mentally Abnormal Offenders*. Cambridge University Press.

Haller, R.M. and Deluty, R.H. (1988) Assaults on staff by psychiatric inpatients – A critical review, *Brit. J. Psychiatr.*, **152**, 174–79.

Jacobs, D. (1983) Evaluation and management of the violent patient in emergency settings. *Psychiatr. Clin. North Am.*, **6**, 259–69.

Kane, J., Honigfeld, G., Singer, J. *et al.* (1988) Clozapine for the Treatment Resistant Schizophrenic. *Arch. Gen. Psychiat.*, **45**, 789–96.

Lerner, Y., Lwow, E., Levitin, A. *et al.* (1979) Acute high-dose parenteral haloperidol treatment of psychosis. *Am. J. Psychiatr.* **36**, 1061–65.

Madden, D.J., Lion, J.R. and Penna, M.W. (1976) Assaults on psychiatrists by patients. *Am. J. Psychiatr.*, **133**, 422–25.

McLaren, S., Browne, F.W.A. and Taylor, P.J. (1990) A study of psychotropic medication given 'as required' in a regional secure unit, *Brit. J. Psychiatr.*, **156**, 732–35.

McNiel, D. and Binder, R. (1989) Relationship between pre-admission threats and later violent behaviour by acute psychiatric inpatients. *Hosp. Comm. Psychiatr.*, **40**, 605–8.

Modell, J.G., Lenox, R.H. and Weiner, S. (1985) Inpatient clinical trial of lorazepam for the treatment of manic agitation. *J. Clin. Psychopharm.*, **5**, 109–13.

Moore, D.P. (1977) Rapid treatment of delirium in critically ill patients. *Am. J. Psychiatr.*, **134**, 1431–2.

Mullen, P. (1988) Violence and mental disorder, *Brit. J. Hosp. Med.*, **40**, 460–63.

Nadelson, T. (1976) The Psychiatrist in the surgical intensive care unit. *Arch. Surg.*, **111**, 113–19.

Neff, K., Denny, D. and Blachly, P. (1972) Control of Severe Agitation with droperidol. *Dis. Nerv. Sys.*, **33**, 594–97.

Noble, P. and Rodgers, S. (1989) Violence by psychiatric inpatients. *Brit. J. Psychiatr.*, **155**, 384–90.

Pearson, M., Wilmot, E. and Padi, M. (1986) A study of violent patients among inpatients in a psychiatric hospital. *Brit. J. Psychiat.*, **149**, 232–35.

Pilowsky, L.S., Ring, H., Shine, P.J. *et al.* (1992) Rapid tranquilisation – a survey of emergency prescribing in a general psychiatric hospital. *Brit. J. Psychiat.* (in press).

Rapp, M.S. (1987) Chemical restraint. *Canadian Journal of Psychiatry*, **32**, 20–21.

Resnick, M. and Burton, B.J. (1984) Droperidol *vs* haloperidol in the initial management of acutely agitated patients. *J. Clin. Psychiatr.*, **45**, 298–99.

Salzman, C. (1988) Use of benzodazepines to control disruptive behaviour in inpatients. *J. Clin. Psychiatr.* **49** (suppl), 13–15.

Schafer, C.B., Shahid, A., Javaid, J.I. *et al.* (1982) Bioavailability of intramuscular versus oral haloperidol in schizophrenic patients. *J. Clin. Pharmacol.*, **2**, 274–77.

Sheard, M.H. (1988) Review: Clinical pharmacology of aggressive behaviour. *Clin. Pharmacol.*, **11**, 483–92.

Tardiff, K., and Sweillam, A. (1980) Assault, suicide and mental illness. *Arch. Gen. Psychiatr.*, **37**, 164–69.

Tesar, G.E., Murray, G.B. and Cassem, N.H. (1985) Use of high-dose intravenous haloperidol in the treatment of agitated cardiac patients. *J. Clin. Psychopharmacol.*, **5**, 344–47.

Tuason, V.B. (1986) A comparison of parenteral loxapine and haloperidol in hostile and aggressive acutely schizophrenic patients, *J. Clin. Psychiatr.*, **47**, 126–29.

Van Putten, T., Marder, S. and Mintz, J. (1990) A controlled dose comparison of haloperidol in newly admitted schizophrenic patients, *Arch. Gen. Psychiatr.*, **47**, 754–58.

Yesavage, J.A. (1982) Inpatient violence and the schizophrenic patient: An inverse correlation between danger-related events and neuroeptic levels, *Biol. Psychiatr.*, **17**, 1331–37.

CHAPTER 10

Coping with violent situations in the caring environment

Andrew McDonnell, John McEvoy and R.L. Dearden

INTRODUCTION

In a recent survey of over 1000 people in the workplace, it was found that 19.6% could recall an incident involving threatening behaviour and 13.5% could recall an actual physical assault (Philips *et al.*, 1989). Yet carers are often surprised when they experience violence from those who are in their care (Owens and Ashcroft, 1985). Health service surveys do not present an optimistic picture; physical assaults can account for as much as 11.5% of all reported incidents; threat with weapons 4.6% and verbal abuse 17% (Health Services Advisory Committee, 1987). Despite these findings comparatively little research is available on how best to manage violent situations in care settings.

In this chapter some of the issues involved in managing violent situations both in community and institutional settings will be examined, with an emphasis on verbal and physical management strategies. Numerous definitions of violence and aggression exist. For the purposes of this chapter the definition made by Blackburn (1988) will be adopted, where violence refers to 'physical acts' and aggression subsumes all verbal behaviours, including threats and physical abuse.

DEFUSING INCIDENTS

Most violent incidents usually have several relatively predictable antecedents. They may be preceded by high levels of arousal and some form of verbal confrontation. Indeed, Luckenbill (1977) suggests that even crimes such as murder can have clear antecedents that build up to the event. In a survey of battered wives, Dobash and Dobash (1984) found that the most common precursor of assault were arguments that led to physical violence. Threatening behaviours are a relatively commonplace occurrence. An example of this was reported by a health visitor in a recent study:

> I was greeted by a very large and irate husband who pushed me against the wall and accused me of not doing enough to help their family.
>
> > (*Philips* et al., *1989*)

This typifies the problems faced by professionals when confronted by hostile clients.

Predicting violent incidents

Stereotypes of victims and offenders permeate society and the media. Lea maintains:

> Entirely random victimization is rare: the crazed gunman who walks down a street shooting at random is not a typical criminal offender. Most offenders have some social or economic relationship to their victims.
>
> > (*Lea, 1992*)

These and other studies imply that there is a certain amount of predictability involved in a violent incident. However, it would be totally incorrect to automatically assume that the 'victim' is to blame for an event. It is similarly erroneous to assume that a 'perpetrator' wanders the streets looking for victims. Clearly, violence is interactional in nature and therefore, it would appear that the predictable aspects of these interactions need to be studied further if the frequency of violent encounters is to be reduced.

The 'assault cycle'

Kaplan and Wheeler (1983) describe a theoretical model that they refer to as the 'assault cycle'. This provides a useful analytical tool for the examination of potentially violent incidents. They describe five phases associated with incidents: (i) the triggering phase; (ii) the escalation phase; (iii) the crisis phase; (iv) the recovery phase; and finally (v) a depression phase that occurs after the crisis. Presumably, if a phase can be recognized then it can be potentially defused. The following section will examine some of the common defusion strategies recommended by researchers.

DEFUSION STRATEGIES

Mood-matching

In normal conversation, people tend to match each other's mood or state of arousal. This concept has been used by some authors when providing advice about the management of aggressive behaviours. For example, if a person is angry and upset and making personal or aggressive comments in a loud voice, an attempt would be made to match the loudness of the voice (arousal level) but not the emotional content or display. Davies (1989) recommends that the carer should attempt to match his or her degree of arousal with the client's. He suggests that: '... one would match the client's aggression with concern, involvement or interest' (Davies, 1989). Similarly, Breakwell (1989) advocates that 'the assailant who shouts, is shouted at: calm intensity is greeted with equal intensity'.

Thus, where 'mood-matching' has been advocated, it is implied that person A attempts to match the person B's arousal but not his or her emotion (Turnbull *et al.*, 1990).

The distinction between matching arousal and not emotional content is quite difficult to grasp and could be potentially very hazardous, particularly if an aggressor perceives an individual as matching both the emotional content and the arousal.

Stewart (1978) advises carers who approach a person who shows signs of becoming aggressive to: '... raise your voice to be heard if the patient is very noisy, but do not give any indications of being aggressive yourself'. This may be difficult. When a person speaks loudly they frequently display nonverbal signs of arousal (Argyle, 1988). Raising one's voice may well help to de-escalate a potentially violent situation, although Davies (1989) admits that it could be potentially dangerous to match aggression with aggression. The authors accept that mood-matching is an attractive option and makes theoretical sense. However, frequently it is not practical and it runs the risk of antagonizing a person who is presumably already highly aroused and possibly dangerous. Furthermore, relatively little is known about the cognitive triggers of violence. One person's aggressive trigger may dampen another person's aggressive intent. For example, social workers are frequently called upon to take both a therapeutic and statutory role when working with families. If a family member is angry or hostile they may 'calm down' when the social worker employs simple 'mood-matching' strategies. However, if the same social worker is required to become involved with the family on a legal or statutory basis, 'mood-matching' approaches may lead to injury or assault because the same social worker is perceived by the family member as a threat.

Low-arousal approaches

Low-arousal approaches are based on the assumption that increases in arousal will most likely result in interpersonal assault. The most often cited principle is to **remain calm** (Department of Health and Social Security, 1976; Confederation of Health Service Employees, 1977; Breakwell, 1989; McDonnell *et al.*, 1991a). This can be achieved by speaking slowly and quietly to the client. An assumption here is that the person who is angry or upset may easily perceive more hostile approaches as threatening. In addition, staff are recommended to breathe normally and to avoid tensing their arms or gritting their teeth (McDonnell *et al.*, 1991a–c).

Nonverbal behaviours

The low-arousal approach has implications for nonverbal as well as verbal behaviours. Direct eye contact is a physiologically arousing phenomenon (Mehrabian, 1972), and prolonged staring at an individual can be interpreted as a signal of attack (Argyle, 1988). Therefore, in the low-arousal approach, eye contact is usually intermittent. To avoid direct eye contact several authors have suggested that a person should stand at a 45° angle from their potential attacker (Davies, 1989; Turnbull *et al.*, 1990).

Low-arousal approaches may have implications for touching people who are angry and/or aroused. Although touching an individual can be a sign of positive communication, aggression is also primarily expressed through bodily contact (Argyle, 1988). Thus touch can be a physiologically arousing phenomenon and it has been recommended that carers should avoid touching clients who are aroused or angry (McDonnell *et al.*, 1991b). Similarly, invading a person's space can be perceived as a threat, therefore potential aggressors should be given a considerable amount of personal space. Kinzel (1970) demonstrated that violent prisoners prefer larger interpersonal spaces than nonviolent prisoners. Turnbull *et al.* (1990) recommended up to '6 m if necessary' in institutional settings.

Posture is another powerful form of nonverbal communication. However, Mehrabian (1969) found that placing your arms on hips is often negatively construed by observers. Some authors recommend placing the hands either in pockets or behind your back. McDonnell *et al.* (1990b) strongly recommend that a carer should adopt a relaxed posture when confronted by an aggressive individual.

Surprise/shock methods

Nonphysical surprise and shock methods are recommended by several authors. To defuse a violent situation Lamplugh (1991) has suggested using one's voice to 'voice off' an attack; '... if you want to give a potential attacker a surprise, expel the air with a bellow or as though you are about to be sick'.

Davies (1990) describes the case of a social worker who witnessed a fight between a father and son on a home visit. He recommended a strategy where the person might have said 'stop hitting him', 'loudly, repeatedly and authoritatively'. These approaches are in almost total contrast to the low-arousal or assertive approaches.

Alarms (either personal or room) are often recommended as an organizational and preventative strategy (Breakwell, 1989). Personal-attack alarms have been proposed presumably for their shock or surprise effect. Lamplugh (1991) proposed that such alarms should be sounded next to the attacker's ear. Presumably this is to surprise, shock or even disable the person. A weakness with this type of approach is when the assailant does not run away – one may then be faced with an aroused, very angry person. Moreover, there are no detailed experimental studies of human responses to the sound of these alarms, although there is a body of research, conducted in New York, that demonstrates the relative difficulty of obtaining bystanders' assistance, even for apparent medical emergencies (Darley and Latane, 1968).

Assertiveness training

Assertiveness has been recommended in a wide range of settings (Rees and Graham, 1991), as an approach to managing aggressive situations, and referred to by some authors as the first line of defence (Davies, 1990). Also it is a relatively popular training option for coping with violence in the workplace (Philips *et al.*, 1989).

The application of assertiveness training to self-protection assumes that people may be attacked or victimized, or are in danger of becoming aggressive themselves, partly because they do not express their wishes, or do so in a socially ineffective manner. As Davies puts it, 'By adopting an assertive attitude, you are telling the world that you are someone to be reckoned with'.

While assertiveness training may help people who are not confident in managing difficult situations, the distinction between assertion and aggression must be appreciated and clearly understood. A drawback of this approach is that people may slip from being assertive to being aggressive. Unfortunately there are few studies of the impact of assertiveness training on people defined as 'high-risk' for violent or aggressive behaviours.

Summary and conclusion

In conclusion, there is a noticeable lack of research evidence for the effectiveness of the defusion strategies discussed in this section.

Some of the strategies mentioned, such as assertiveness training and low-arousal approaches, appear to make some intuitive sense. Strategies that are based on surprise or shock and to a certain extent 'mood-matching' appear to be a little more risky to the individual because they may have unpredictable consequences and encourage a fight and flight reaction. Some of the advice is not only contradictory (e.g. 'mood-matching' versus low-arousal approaches) but, in some cases, dangerous. Surprise and shock methods would appear to be useful only in cases of severe desperation. Much more research is needed to assess the relative merits of these strategies before firm conclusions can be drawn or clear advice given to carers. In the following section, the use of some of the more invasive methods recommended for dealing with aggression and violence will be examined.

RESTRAINT PROCEDURES

The lack of an adequate definition of physical restraint (Dabrowski *et al.*, 1986) makes consideration of the literature problematic. For the purposes of this chapter, the term physical restraint refers to, 'the restraint of an individual by the use of bodily force'. Mechanical restraint will refer to 'restraint that involves the use of devices that are physically attached to the person', such as protective splints, leather straps, etc. There is evidence that such procedures are used in a variety of care settings.

Physical restraint

A survey of Polish psychiatric facilities reported that physical restraint was used in over 30% of acute admissions (Dabrowski *et al.*, 1986). This rather high figure is accounted for by a broad definition of physical restraint, which included forced feeding, medication and the use of mechanical restraints. In a survey of a US hospital-based neurosurgical unit, physical restraint was employed in over 35% of cases of cerebral contusions (Edlund *et al.*, 1991). The authors found that 'restrained' individuals tended to be prescribed psychotropic drugs frequently during their stay in hospital and tended to have consumed alcohol prior to admission.

Physical restraint is commonly used in settings for the elderly, with figures varying between 25% and 84.6% (Evans and Strumpf, 1989). It has been employed with violent adolescents (Hunter, 1989) and in a recent study of carers of people with learning difficulties, physical restraint was used as a management strategy in 20% of incidents (McDonnell and McEvoy, in press).

Side-effects

The use of physical restraint can have serious side-effects on care staff. It is believed that most staff-related injuries in psychiatric settings are restraint- or seclusion-related (Haller and Deluty, 1988). In a study of staff injuries in a US Mental Handicap Service it was found that 29.5% of staff injuries could be attributed to the implementation of mechanical or physical restraint (Hill and Spreat, 1987). Physical restraint can also lead to the injury of clients (Dietz and Rada, 1983; Spreat and Baker-Potts, 1983).

Difficulties in using physical restraint

Although most surveys on the incidence and effects of restraint procedures suffer from a variety of methodological problems, the evidence suggests that physical restraint procedures are still widely used in a variety of caring environments. Yet there has been surprisingly little research into the effectiveness of various types of restraint procedures. Most methods appear to have developed without any experimental evidence for their effectiveness. Some procedures recommend two members of staff should carry out procedures (Harvey and Schepers, 1979; Lefensky *et al.* 1978; McDonnell *et al.*, 1991c), others suggest as many as four staff (Lion *et al.*, 1972; Reid, 1973). Often there is a lack of consensus over the restraint procedures themselves. Fidone (1988) referred to the problems of applying a 'baskethold' on clients in a supine position. In a reply Steinfield (1988) pointed out that the 'baskethold' was only applied in a prone position. If restraint is to be used, then the confusion surrounding terminology requires attention and the procedures need the utmost scrutiny, for the protection of both clients and care staff.

Mechanical restraint

Most of the published information reviewed here is from studies in the USA. There is little information about UK practices, although it is clear that mechanical restraints are sometimes used. They have been advocated for violent individuals in a variety of care settings (Evans and Strumpf, 1989; Van Rybroek *et al.*, 1987). A major problem with the literature is defining what types of devices are used. Mattresses (Penningroth, 1975) and blankets (Powers, 1987) have been recommended. Anders (1983) described a restraint method that involved a person being strapped to a bed in a supine position by use of leather straps. More recently the 'cold wet sheet pack' is reportedly still being employed in some institutions (Ross *et al.*, 1988). This is a procedure commonly used in the early part of the 20th century, which involved wrapping people in cold, wet sheets. This allegedly had powerful sedative effects. Some physical restraint procedures involve the 'locking' of limbs, which, in effect, involves using pain to control a violent individual. An apparently new approach has been the adoption of preventative ambulatory devices (PADs) (Van Rybroek *et al.*, 1987) as an alternative to seclusion. This method involves the application of either wrist and/or ankle restraints, which have a remarkable similarity to 'handcuffs and shackles'.

Effective and acceptable?

McDonnell and Sturmey (1993) have argued that the effectiveness of a restraint procedure is only one useful measure and the social validation of these methods must be addressed. A recent study asked a sample of young people to rate videotaped representations of three commonly used restraint procedures using the *Treatment Evaluation Inventory* (McDonnell *et al.*, 1993; McDonnell and McEvoy, in press). Two of the methods involved restraining a person on the floor, the third restraining a client in an armchair. It was found that all of the samples rated 'the chair method' as more socially acceptable. It is difficult to generalize to all care settings from the results of this study and clearly more research is needed before advocating the use of a single method. This highlights a methodology for investigating the acceptability of physical restraint procedures and verbal strategies for managing incidents. How procedures would be viewed by the public is just as important as their effectiveness. How would members of the public and care staff rate the acceptability of shouting at individuals even if it were an extremely effective strategy?

Staff training in restraint methods

A neglected area of research is the training and evaluation of care staff in physical-management procedures. A survey of 67 psychiatric nurses found that 75% had received no training in the prevention and management of disturbed behaviour (Basque and Merhige, 1980). A few studies have reported some evaluations of training. In a comparison of trained versus untrained staff in a state psychiatric hospital it was found that there were fewer reports of assault on staff who had received training (Infantino and Musingo, 1983; Whittington and Wykes, 1993) although others (e.g. Roscoe, 1987) have shown that trained staff are more likely to be included in violent incidents.

Gertz (1980) described the effects of a 2-day workshop taught to 317 staff members in a mental health centre. They found a reduction in patient-related accidents from 174 incidents to 117. Turnbull (personal communication) reported increases in self-confidence and performances of care staff who attended a 2-week residential training course. More recently, McDonnell (in press) found increases in confidence scores of care staff who attended a 3-day workshop in the management of violent and aggressive behaviours. Staff skills in the use of a two-person restraint procedure were assessed by means of a videotaped role-play test. No studies to date have reported adequate follow-up data, and many of the studies have failed to include treatment control groups or measures of generalization of skills to the workplace. Future research studies might examine usefully the effect training in the restraint procedures might have on the reduction of staff injuries. Evaluation of staff training might also consider the extent to which staff are encouraged to feel more confident and able to cope with violent situations. In a study carried out by Whittington and Wykes (1993) a 1-day violence course using role play reduced levels of violence on wards but only when a significant number of staff from a ward had attended.

Seclusion

The seclusion of an individual involves his or her isolation in a designated locked area. Seclusion is frequently recommended for the protection of staff and clients from assault and for a decrease in sensory or emotional input (Hodgkinson, 1985). This emotional input may be in the form of negative interactions with staff or clients, or merely providing a quiet area for the person (Gutheil, 1978). However, it has been argued that there is no clear theoretical rationale for the use of seclusion (Drinkwater and Gudjonsson, 1989).

Difficulties in implementing seclusion

Several studies have reported difficulties with the implementation of seclusion. It may be used for a large number of behaviours and not only in cases of violence and may also be used more frequently in some institutions than others. Hodgkinson (1985) found that the most common reported use of seclusion was for general disturbed behaviour rather than violence *per se*. Carpenter *et al*. (1988), in a survey of 19 hospitals in New York State, found that city and large-town hospitals used seclusion more than suburban and small-town hospitals. In a study of a UK psychiatric unit, high usage of seclusion was associated with lower staffing levels and less experienced staff in charge of the ward (Morrison and LeRoux, 1987).

Seclusion practices raise several questions. Has training been provided to care staff as to how to move a violent individual into an area designated for seclusion and what form does this training take? The utility of seclusion can be questioned because it arouses negative imagery associated with imprisonment. Furthermore, recent evidence suggests that psychiatric services can apparently manage without the use of these methods (Kingdon and Bakewell, 1988). The role of seclusion in UK special hospitals has been called into question and is now the subject of a proposed national governmental inquiry.

SELF-DEFENCE TRAINING

Although no accurate surveys exist it appears that self-defence classes are quite a popular option in the UK. In their discussion of violence in the workplace, Philips *et al.* (1989) reported that self-defence classes were being introduced into worksettings and appeared to be popular with the 'youngest and oldest age groups'. Moreover, brief courses aimed at teaching essential combative skills are most certainly being taught to members of the caring services. The Department of Health and Social Security report entitled *'Violence to Staff'* gave an opinion about the use of self-defence techniques:

> Some authorities arrange self-defence classes for their staff of both sexes. We do not make such a recommendation ourselves. Although the boost to confidence is important, we are of the view that elementary self-defence techniques have little practical value in a real-life incident and might cause harm to the assailant or expose the victim to more serious injury.
>
> *(DHSS, 1988)*

Despite these warnings, it appears that self-defence training is an option for managing violent incidents in the caring services. GPs, social workers, midwives etc. often have to make home visits to areas that may have a high frequency of street crime. A distinction has to be made between an assault on a carer by a member of the public 'on the street' and the carer who is working in that capacity with a client in a caring context. While the law states that an individual may use 'reasonable force' to defend themselves if attacked, it is difficult to define operationally what is meant by the term **reasonable**. A person who defends themselves during a mugging may be able to argue that the vicious blows and techniques employed were in self-defence. However, a person working in a caring environment could be subject to dismissal for similar behaviour in the care setting. Several staff have gone to prison for assaults on clients despite using a self-defence argument (Martin, 1984).

Gaining confidence

Although a popular growth industry in the UK, there is little evidence for the efficacy of self-defence training. Pava *et al.* (1991) reported on the effectiveness of self-defence training for a group of 11 visually impaired women. The course consisted of 12 2-hour sessions, involving physical resistance skills, rape prevention strategies and the discussion and rehearsal of 'rape scenarios'. The authors reported significant increases in the confidence women placed in the strategies they were taught and a statistically significant increase in the women's reported confidence in their ability to respond to a threatening situation. The authors reported post-test improvements in the physical skills taught on the course. However, the study did not include a control group and no follow-up measures were taken; despite these weaknesses the study is praiseworthy in its attempt to measure the effectiveness of such training.

An increase in self-confidence has been reported by researchers who have conducted staff-training courses containing physical self-defence components. Turnbull *et al.* (1990) found that most staff who completed a 2-week training course that included physical skills reported feeling more confident, although no data were presented. McDonnell (in press) reported increases in a pre- and post-test self-confidence scale following a 3-day training course for care staff in facilities for people with learning difficulties. Over 50% of this course involved the teaching of physical skills drawn from the martial art of Jiu-Jitsu and modified for the caring environment. Both Turnbull *et al.* (1990) and McDonnell (in press) used role play; a method recommended for use in self-defence classes (McGrath and Tegner, 1977).

Learning techniques and skills

The pop singer Lynsey DePaul (1992) has recently produced a short self-defence training video for women containing 19 different self-defence techniques, ranging from being grabbed by the wrist, to being pinned to the floor. It is difficult to comprehend how a person could master so many motor skills in such a short period of time, simply from video presentation. An analogy here would be to expect a person to learn to be a rock climber or drive a car as a direct result of watching and practising from a video. To some extent this video package is characteristic of the brief and extremely violent nature of self-defence procedures.

The problem of teaching and learning, at times quite complex, motor skills is not only unique to video recordings. The first author (a UK National Coach in the martial art of Jiu-Jitsu) reviewed a selection of books on self-defence. A review by the first author and Steven Alison (a member of the British Jiu-Jitsu Association) of books on self-defence published in Britain is shown in Table 10.1. A similar pattern to that found in video packages emerges, with a vast number of physical skills being described and visually displayed. These books comprise a

Table 10.1 An analysis of the numbers of physical techniques recommended in a selection of UK self-defence books

	Number of pages	Number of physical techniques	Percentage of book
Streetwise: A Basic Guide to Self Defence (Lowe et al., 1984)	112	25	22
Self Defence for Women (Warren-Holland et al., 1987)	140	29	21
Hit Back: Self Defence for Women (Biffen and Search, 1983)	176	60	34
Protect Yourself: Every Woman's Survival Course (Whitelaw, 1985)	159	47	29
Hands Off: Hapkido Self Defence for Women (Adams and Webster, 1986)	95	29	30
The Official Self-Defence Handbook (Mitchell, 1985)	152	45	29
Protect Yourself: A Woman's Handbook (Davies, 1990)	160	23	14
Stand Your Ground: A Woman's Guide to Self Preservation (Quinn, 1983)	175	50	29

large number of pages on physical procedures even though it is unclear whether an individual is expected to learn these skills from the books on their own. Many of these techniques appear to be extremely violent in nature and the books include very little information on defusing violent situations. Lamplugh (1991) has cogently argued that '... techniques are almost impossible to learn from books, they need hands-on training and to be regularly practised'. However, Lamplugh later recommends in the same book: '... try twisting the ears off' and 'bend any finger right back (not just a little way). Stamp on them, bite them, pull them apart'. Of even more concern is the fact that accurate studies have not been undertaken into the maintenance and generalization of self-defence skills taught in evening classes throughout the UK.

Difficulties with self-defence training

It may be misguided to assume that relatively short self-defence courses will have major effects on human behaviour, although it would appear logical (but requiring much more empirical research) that self-defence training can increase an individual's confidence in managing a violent encounter and make that person more aware of preventative strategies. However, a major difficulty with self-defence based training is how it relates to the caring environment, especially the concerns about the content of such training. A preoccupation with violent and potentially lethal physical techniques seems to abound. Paul (1980) expressed concerns that self-defence class instructors appeared to be imparting potentially dangerous techniques. This finding is of particular concern when coupled with research indicating a negative relationship between skill level and aggressiveness (Nosanchuk, 1981). Theoretically, short courses could conceivably teach quite high levels of aggressive response to people with comparatively poor skill levels.

Are the procedures taught effective as well as socially acceptable? Does the person teaching the course have any experience of working with the client groups concerned? Are these instructors suitably qualified? Unfortunately the national guidelines on self-defence training are sufficiently vague to allow a frightening degree of variability in training and teaching competence. The growth industry associated with self-defence training requires a high degree of scrutiny and systematic research by members of the caring service. Its introduction to the care environment is fraught with dangers and, at present, leaves too many important questions unanswered.

GENERAL CONCLUSION

Simple answers to the provision of coping with violence in caring environments are not available, since many of the issues associated with the management of violent incidents in the care setting are multicomplex. Research into the strategies of managing these behaviours is woefully inadequate. The defusion strategies frequently recommended are sometimes contradictory, may in themselves prompt aggression and require careful consideration. Where physical procedures, such as restraint or seclusion are used, it is imperative that staff are trained in their usage and considerable investigation into the social acceptability of these methods is undertaken prior to implementation.

A further aspect worthy of systematic investigation is the viewpoint of the consumer. How socially acceptable to persons who are at risk of committing aggression are the procedures employed against them? To date, there appears to be little research into this interesting avenue of enquiry. How would people respond to the question, 'what do you think of how you were secluded or restrained?'?

The need for staff training

Guidelines or a 'blueprint' for good staff training in the management of violence are lacking. Ideally, training courses might include aspects of environmental design, diffusion strategies and simple relatively non-violent methods of managing incidents. It appears to make intuitive sense that a person needs to feel confident if they are to defuse success-fully a potentially violent incident. It is more likely that this confidence will be engendered if the person has had training in the prediction of violent incidents and the social skills training for defusing incidents, as well as dealing with the physical consequences of violent acts and the consequences of their own physical behaviour. This is true whether training involves restraint procedures, or exposure to simple physical skills in order to help the person escape from the situation. Concen-trating on one aspect or another would appear to be only half the answer.

The need for research

In conclusion, the research on managing violent incidents especially in UK care settings is sparse, imprecise and confusing. Advice for carers on how to defuse and physically manage violent situations in caring environments is given with a confidence based on very shaky founda-tions. Most of this advice is based on anecdotal information and gives licence to the frequent employment of violent interventions in com-munity and particularly institutional settings.

Physical solutions as responses to crises may appear to be sufficient in the short-term. However, such solutions frequently have negative side-effects in the long-term. Only when there is open and frank discussion of the complex issues involved, clarification of definitions and the systematic description of procedures undertaken will signifi-cant progress be made. Training care staff would appear to be a necessity; however, the content of the training is yet to be decided and is still a question of considerable debate. There needs to be more research data and fewer anecdotes in this field. Perhaps this could be achieved through anonymous data collection across UK care settings so that at least an overview of the types of physical techniques used could be catalogued.

REFERENCES

Adams, F. and Webster, G. (1986) *Hands Off: Hapkido Self Defence for Women*, Jarrolds, Norwich.

Anders, R. (1983) Management of violent patients. *Critical Care Update*, 41–47.

Argyle, M. (1988) *Bodily Communication*, Methuen, London.

Basque, L.O., and Merhige, J. (1980) Nurses' experience with dangerous behaviour: Implication for training. *Journal of Continuing Education in Nursing*, **11**, 47–50.

Biffen, C., and Search, G. (1983) *Hit Back: Self Defence for Women*. Fontana, Glasgow.

Blackburn, R. (1988), Cognitive behavioural approaches to understanding and treating aggression, in *Clinical Approaches to Violence*, (eds K. Howells and C. Hollin), John Wiley, Chichester.

Breakwell, G. (1989) *Facing Physical Violence*, Routledge, London.

Carpenter, M.D., Hannon, V.R., McCleery, G. *et al.* (1988) Variations in seclusion and restraint practices by hospital location. *Hospital and Community Psychiatry*, **39**, 418–23.

Confederation of Health Service Employees (COHSE) (1977) *The Management of Violent or Potentially Violent Patients. Report Of A Special Working Party Offering Information, Advice and Guidance to COHSE Members*. COHSE, London.

Dabrowski, S., Frydman, L. and Azkowska-Dabrowska, T. (1986) Physical restraint in Polish psychiatric facilities. *International Journal of Law and Psychiatry*, **8**, 369–82.

Darley, J.M. and Latane, B. (1968) Bystander intervention in emergencies: Diffusion of responsibility. *Journal of Personality and Social Psychology*, **8**, 377–83.

Davies, J. (1990). *Protect Yourself!: A Womans Handbook*. London: Piatkus.

Davies, W. (1989) The Prevention of Assault on Professional Helpers, in *Clinical Approaches to Violence*, (Eds K. Howells and C.R. Hollin), John Wiley, Chichester.

Department of Health and Social Security (1976) *The Management of Violent or Potentially Violent Hospital Patients*. Health Circular HC (76)11, HMSO, London.

Department of Health and Social Security (1988) *Violence to Staff*. Report of the DHSS Advisory Committee on Violence to Staff. HMSO, London.

De Paul, L. (1992) *Taking Control: Basic Mental and Physical Self Defence for Women*. (video) Polygram, London.

Dietz, P.E. and Rada, R.T. (1983) Interpersonal violence in forensic facilities, in *Assaults within Psychiatric Facilities*, (eds J.R. Lion and W.H. Reid), Grune and Stratton, New York.

Dobash, R.E. and Dobash, R.P. (1984) The nature and antecedents of violent events. *British Journal of Criminology*, **24**, 268–88.

Drinkwater, J. and Gudjonsson, G.H. (1989) The nature of violence in psychiatric hospitals, in *Clinical Approaches to Violence*. (eds K. Howells and C.R. Hollin), John Wiley, Chichester.

Edlund, M.J., Goldberg, R.J. and Morris, P.L. (1991) The use of physical restraint in patients with cerebral contusion. *International Journal of Psychiatry in Medicine*, **21**, 173–82.

Evans, L.K. and Strumpf, N.E. (1989) Tying down the elderly: A review of the literature on physical restraint. *Journal of the American Geriatrics Society*, **37**, 65–74.

Fidone, G.S. (1988) Risks in physical restraint. *Hospital and Community Psychiatry*, **39**, 203.

Gertz, B. (1980) Training for prevention of assaultive behaviour in a psychiatric setting. *Hospital and Community Psychiatry*, **31**, 628–30.

Gutheil, T. (1978) Observations on the theoretical basis for seclusion of the psychiatric in patient. *American Journal of Psychiatry*, **135**, 325–28.

Haller, R.M. and Deluty, R.H. (1988) Assaults on staff by psychiatric in-patients: A critical review. *British Journal of Psychiatry*, **152**, 174–79.

Harvey, E.R. and Schepers, J. (1977) Physical control techniques and defensive holds for use with aggressive retarded adults. *Mental Retardation*, **15**, 29–31.

Health Services Advisory Committee (1987) *Violence to Staff in the Health Services*, Health and Safety Commission, London.

Hodgkinson, P. (1985) The use of seclusion. *Medical Science and Law*, **25**, 215–22.

Hill, J. and Spreat, S. (1987) Staff injury rates associated with the implementation of contingent restraint. *Mental Retardation*, **25**, 141–45.

Hunter, D.S. (1989) The use of physical restraint in managing out of control behaviour in youth: A frontline perspective. *Child and Youth Care Quarterly*, **18**, 141–54.

Infantino, J.A. and Musingo, S.Y. (1983) Assaults and injuries among staff with and without aggression control techniques. *Hospital and Community Psychiatry*, **36**, 1312–14.

Kaplan, S.G. and Wheeler, E.G. (1983) Survival skills for working with potentially violent clients. *Social Casework*, **64**, 339–45.

Kingdon, D.E. and Bakewell, E.W. (1988) Aggressive behaviour: Evaluation of a nonseclusion policy of a district psychiatric service. *British Journal of Psychiatry*, **153**, 631–34.

Kinzel, A.F. (1970) Body buffer zones in violent prisoners. *American Journal of Psychiatry*, **127**, 59–64.

Lamplugh, D. (1991) *Without Fear: The Key to Staying Safe*, Weidenfeld and Nicolson, London.

Lea, J. (1992). The analysis of crime, in *Rethinking Criminology: The Realist Debate*, (eds J. Young and R. Mathews), Sage, London.

Lefensky, B., DePalma, T. and Lociercero, D. (1978) Management of violent behaviours. *Perspectives in Psychiatric Care*, **16**, 212–17.

Lion, J.R., Levenberg, L.B. and Strong, R.E. (1972) Restraining the violent patient. *Journal of Psychiatric Nursing and Mental Health Services*, **32**, 497–98.

Lowe, J., Wright, I. and Finn, M. (1984) *Streetwise: A Basic Guide to Self Defence*, Ariel Books, London.

Luckenbill, D.F. (1977) Criminal homicide as a situated transaction. *Social Problems*, **25**, 176–86.

McDonnell, A.A. (in press) Training care staff to manage violent incidents: A report on a 3-day training course, (paper submitted for publication).

McDonnell, A.A. and McEvoy, J. (in press) Care staff perceptions of the topography of physically aggressive behaviours in persons with a learning difficulty, (paper submitted for publication).

McDonnell, A.A., and Sturmey, P.S. (1993) Managing violent and aggressive behaviour: towards a better practice, in *Challenging Behaviours and People with Learning Difficulties: A Psychological Perspective*, (eds R.S.P. Jones and C. Eayrs), British Institute of Learning Disabilities, Kidderminster.

McDonnell, A.A., Dearden, R. and Richens, A. (1991a) Staff training in the management of violence and aggression: 1. Setting up a training system. *Mental Handicap*, **19**, 73–76.

McDonnell, A.A., Dearden, R. and Richens, A. (1991b) Staff training in the management of violence and aggression: 2. Avoidance and escape principles. *Mental Handicap*, **19**, 109–12.

McDonnell, A.A., Dearden, R. and Richens, A. (1991c) Staff training in the management of violence and aggression: 3. Physical restraint procedures. *Mental Handicap*, **19**, 151–54.

McDonnell, A.A., Sturmey, P.S. and Dearden, R.L. (1993) The acceptability of physical restraint procedures. *Behavioural and Cognitive Psychotherapy*, **21**(3), 255–64.

McGrath, A. and Tegner, B. (1977) Co-educational self defence. *Journal of Physical Education Research*, **42**, 28–29.

Martin, J.P. (1984) *Hospitals in Trouble*, Blackwell, Oxford.

Mehrabian, A. (1969) Significance of posture and position in the communication of attitude and status relationships. *Psychological Bulletin*, **71**, 359–72.

Mehrabian, A. (1972) *Nonverbal Communication*, Aldine-Atherton, Chicago and New York.

Mitchell, D. (1985) *The Official Self-defence Handbook*, Pelham, London.

Morrison, P. and LeRoux, B. (1987) The practice of seclusion. *Nursing Times*, **83**, 62–66.

Nosanchuk, T.A. (1981) The way of the warrior: The effects of traditional martial arts training on aggressiveness. *Human Relations*, **34**, 435–44.

Owens, R.G. and Ashcroft, J.B. (1985) *Violence: A Guide for the Caring Professions*, Croom Helm, Dover.

Paul, W.W. (1980) Aggression control and non verbal communication: Aspects of Asian martial arts. *Dissertation Abstracts International*, **40**, 5873.

Pava, W.S., Bateman, P., Appleton, M.K. *et al.* (1991) Self-defence training for visually impaired women. *Journal of Visual Impairment and Blindness*, **32**, 397–401.

Penningroth, P. (1975) Control of violence in a mental health setting. *American Journal of Nursing*, **75**, 606–9.

Philips, C.M., Stockdale, J.E. and Joeman, L. (1989) *The Risks In Going To Work: The Naure of People's Work, The Risks They Encounter and the Incidence of Sexual Harassment, Physical Attack and Threatening Behaviour*, Suzy Lamplugh Trust, London.

Powers, T. (1987) Professional survival tips: Defensive tactics for dealing with the uncooperative patient. *Peripatetic Nursing Quarterly*, **3**, 59–66.

Quinn, K. (1983) *Stand Your Ground*, Orbis, London.

Rees, S. and Graham, R.S. (1991) *Assertion Training: How To Be Who You Really Are*. Routledge, London.

Reid, J.A. (1973) Controlling the fight/flight patient. *Canadian Nurse*, **69**, 30–34.

Roscoe, J. (1987) *Survey on Incidence and Nature of Violence*. Report to Working Party on Violence, Bethlem, Royal and Maudsley Hospitals Special Health Authority, London.

Ross, D.R., Lewin, R., Gold, K. *et al.* (1988) The psychiatric uses of cold, wet sheet packs. *American Journal of Psychiatry*, **145**, 242–45.

Spreat, S. and Baker-Potts, J.C. (1983) Patterns of injury in institutionalized residents. *Mental Retardation*, **21**, 23–29.

Steinfield, J. (1988) Physical restraint. *Hospital and Community Psychiatry*, **39**, 788.

Stewart, A.T. (1978) Handling the aggressive patient. *Perspectives in Psychiatric Care*, **16**, 212–17.

Turnbull, J., Aitken, I., Black, L. *et al.* (1990) Turn it around: Short-term management for aggression and anger. *Journal of Psychosocial Nursing*, **28**, 8–11.

Turnbull, J. personal communication.

Van Rybroek, G.J., Kuhlman, T.L., Maier, G.J. *et al.* (987) Preventative Aggression Devices (PADS): Ambulatory restraints as an alternative to seclusion. *The Journal of Psychiatry*, **48**, 401–5.

Warren-Holland, D., Russell-Jones, D. and Stewart, R. (1987) *Self Defence for Women*, Hamlin, Twickenham.

Whitelaw, J. (1985) *Protect Yourself: Every Woman's Survival Guide*, Javelin Books, Poole.

Whittington, R. and Wykes, T. (1993) Evaluation of a training package for staff working with violent psychiatric patients. Unpublished manuscript.

CHAPTER 11

Counselling for victims of violence

Til Wykes and Gillian Mezey

INTRODUCTION

Work, like the home, is regarded as a safe place and yet iron-ically individuals in both settings are at a greater risk of violence than in the community (Brodsky, 1976; Mezey and Rubenstein, 1992).

Violence at work is often not conceptualized by the victim as a crime; it appears a matter of private and personal rather than public concern. Thus the victim seeks to remedy the problem through alterations in inter- and intrapersonal relationships rather than seeking a more public remedy outside the institution in which he or she operates. Many individuals also experience a secondary victimization due to the unsympathetic or unsupportive reactions of the immediate social network (Silverman, 1978).

When someone is attacked or threatened in the workplace they experience psychological sequelae similar to victims of other personal assaults. These psychological 'symptoms' are not abnormal but are normal responses to abnormal circumstances. They include anger, guilt, shame, humiliation, sleep difficulties, depression, anxiety, hyper-vigilance, suspiciousness, increased arousal and phobias. Further details of these symptoms are given in Chapter 8.

The reactions may be shortlived but they may also be made worse by several factors. The individual's available coping strategies affect the overall response; the work environment may also have an effect. Often nonaffected individuals in an organization blame the victim for his or her involvement in the incident or protect themselves by evolving the view that it was something in the victim's personality that produced the violent encounter. Together with the response by the manage-ment of the organization, these factors will affect the victim's ability to survive a violent encounter.

Although there are similarities between crime victims and people who are the victims of violence at work there are also differences. For instance, the organizational response has an effect on the psychological difficulties experienced. Colleagues, in particular, can have a dramatic effect on the victim's experiences. These effects are equivalent to the secondary victimization experienced by the victims of crime where it is the result of unsympathetic reactions from the police and the criminal justice system. However, these people are rarely familiar and trusted members of an individual's social network and, although there are undoubtedly effects on crime victims from their close friends and relatives, the effect of being blamed and/or unsupported by colleagues must add a further dimension to victimization at work.

Apart from the differences in secondary victimization there is also the nature of the work itself that changes responses. When crime victims know their assailants the reactions are worse. In the caring professions the victim nearly always knows the assailant and, in addition, is often providing a service to them that usually involves some support. The violence therefore violates several assumptions about the work role and the competence of the individual who has chosen to work in a profession that requires so much human contact.

The closely knit communities within the caring professions also have traditional rules of conduct and so it is counter-cultural to admit to feeling like a victim. Caregivers have an image of being strong and in control and this sometimes leads to difficulties in coming to terms with the psychological reactions of being a victim.

The provision of treatment also has its negative connotations. Treatment is given to those who are not self-sufficient and the term itself may reinforce the lowered self-image of many employee victims.

These factors all affect the response and the sensitive provision of care following violence at work. However, in order to be able to intervene a working model of the underlying processes that support the psychological reactions is needed. The following are some of the models that have been suggested.

MODELS OF STRESS RESPONSES

Crisis theory

Caplan (1964) describes 'crisis' as a 'state of psychological disequilibrium that may last for a period of about 6 weeks'. Individuals inevitably have to adapt following any crisis and the presence of appropriate coping behaviours in response to an assault, representing a crisis, will lead to either mastery or to failure (Lindeman, 1944). A crucial aspect of crisis counselling is to reinvest the victim with a sense of control, while at the same time discouraging excess dependency on the therapist. People who have experienced violence or threats would feel dependent, unable to find or order information as a direct result of the stressor and so their main need is for pastoral care in which the responsibility for immediate decisions is taken by others (especially as the cognitive capacity of the victim is likely to be affected).

Bereavement

Many authors and victims have likened the psychological responses to violence at work to the reactions following bereavement (BASW, 1988; Ochberg, 1988). Violence may, in itself, be experienced as a series of multiple losses – loss of self identity, sense of invulnerability and control, as well as the physical incapacity resulting from the more serious acts of violence. Certainly there are several similar features to bereavement in the processes of realization, alarm, re-experiencing and regaining control or re-equilibration. Bereavement is a normal and painful emotional state that follows the loss of a loved one. The therapeutic endeavour is to allow the expression of affect, to understand the meaning of the incident, to elucidate ambivalence about it and to free the event of its uncontrollable painful emotional recollections (Parkes, 1975).

These therapeutic aims are important in dealing with employee victims but there are several differences relating mainly to the victimization of the individual. For example, whereas the bereaved person experiences the loss of a significant other, the victim of violence at work is harmed or coerced by another person. The bereaved person has a feeling of loss and a profound feeling of sadness but the employee victim feels like a loser and is humiliated. Finally, the bereaved people feel that part of themselves has gone but the employee victims feel let down, exploited and invaded. The therapist's goal is to explain the differences between bereavement and these psychological consequences of violence and to normalize them. The therapist can also help the employee victim to understand the reasons for the ostracism and blame, while disagreeing with those who perpetuate it.

Arousal

The high arousal experienced after a violent incident drives several of the symptoms, for example hyperalertness, startle responses, etc. In the absence of the feared stimulus, it may also produce symptoms of anxiety such as panic and the development of phobias. This high level of anxiety can be dealt with by systematic desensitization but there are cases that will not respond to this sort of therapy. Pharmacotherapy can be useful, particularly to alleviate the chronic symptoms of hyperarousal (Davidson, 1992; Van der Kolk, 1987). However, many of these drugs also carry unwanted and potentially dangerous side-effects, which can be handicapping and distressing to the individual in the long term.

Post-traumatic responses

The reactions of victims of all sorts of traumas are very similar and have been recognized by being given a separate diagnostic classification – post-traumatic stress disorder (PTSD: DSMIIIr; American Psychiatric Association, 1987). The disorder consists of three main types of symptoms and encompasses ingredients of all the other three models already suggested. These are symptoms of high arousal, avoidance and re-experiencing. The symptoms of post-traumatic stress response are:

1. High arousal:
   (a) Irritability
   (b) Difficulty falling asleep
   (c) Startle response;
2. Avoidance:
   (a) Numbness
   (b) Avoiding situations or people who remind you of the event;
3. Re-experiencing (e.g. flashbacks).

Mowrer's two-factor theory invokes both instrumental and classical conditioning to account for the creation and perpetuation of post-traumatic stress disorder (Mowrer, 1947). A previously neutral stimulus such as patient contact (conditioned stimulus) becomes paired with a threatening assault (unconditioned stimulus), resulting in a fear response. The conditioned stimulus (CS) of patient contact then becomes capable of eliciting a conditioned fear response (CR). This conditioned fear response may then generalize to associated stimuli, such as the ward, the hospital or professional colleagues. The second stage of the process involves a reinforcement of fear-induced avoidance behaviour by a resulting decrease in anxiety levels, which encourages further avoidance.

Edna Foa and colleagues (Foa and Kozak, 1986; Foa *et al.*, 1989) have extended this theoretical formulation to produce a model on which to base therapeutic interventions. They proposed that 'fear is represented in memory structures that serve as blueprints for fear behaviour and therapy is a process by which these structures are modified' (Foa and Kozak, 1986, p. 21). In their model, emotions are represented as information structures in memory. Anxiety occurs when an information structure that serves as a programme to escape or avoid danger is activated. The fear structure contains information about the feared stimuli and behavioural and physiological responses as well as cognitive attributions (or interpretive information) about the meaning of the events represented in the fear structure. This last sort of information is essential because there must be some way of representing danger in the structure. For example, the stimulus and response information contained in a programme for running around a track ahead of a baton-carrying competitor is the same as for running in front of a club-carrying assailant. What is different about the two situations is the meaning of the event.

In order to intervene to change the fear structure it must first be activated then elements must be presented that are incompatible with elements present in the structure. This new information has to be integrated into the evoked-information structure for an emotional change to take place. For example, in the case of a simple phobia of dogs, the fear structure is activated by exposure to the feared stimulus – a dog. Information about some dogs not being dangerous is presented and the new memory of this information, which contains both cognitive and emotional elements, should then be incorporated before the fear can be diminished. In PTSD, the fear structures contain many elements because of the strength of the traumatic event. Following a trauma, many stimuli and responses that had previously signalled safety are now associated with danger and because few stimuli can now act as safety signals in the environment, the individual is in a state of constant fear.

Fear structures become activated when elements in them match elements in the real world. Since these structures are so large in PTSD, elements are often matched and therefore the structures themselves often become activated producing frequent bursts of arousal (e.g. startle). These may alternate with avoidance responses (e.g. numbness). This activation may account for the overwhelming number of fear experiences reported by PTSD sufferers and the disruption to their daily lives. Problems for therapy include trying to match all elements because of the large size of the fear structure. The structure may also be more difficult to access as a whole and may not always be completely activated.

The fear structures of people who experience violence at work may be of varying sizes and have varying elements laid down depending on several issues. For instance, individuals will differ in their prior assumptions about the world, their safety signals, the nature of the incident, its perception and the level of arousal produced. Each person's symptoms will be dependent on the matching of elements in their own individual fear structures and so a range of reactions in this group of victims will be produced.

These theories of the representation and interaction of cognitive, physiological and emotional processes were originally formulated to describe phobias and they have since been generalized to PTSD. This generalization has only involved postulating an increased size and potency to the fear structure and if this is the only change needed then one could propose a range of fear structures that are built up in response to events that may not necessarily meet the DSMIIIr criteria for trauma (Chapter 6). Events that include violence or threats could therefore be seen as destroying prior safety assumptions (and are therefore unpredictable) and enabling the creation of fear structures, which could produce a range of symptomatic outcomes.

Neurobiological models of PTSD

These neurobiological models (Van der Kolk *et al.*, 1985; Giller 1990) are based on the animal model of 'inescapable shock' and the effects on neurotransmitter activity in the brain, in particular, catecholamine depletion and stress-induced analgesia. If one were to accept a neurobiological basis for the disorder then this implies that treatments should correct neurotransmitter imbalance. So far, the trials of the effectiveness of medication have been disappointingly inconclusive (Davidson *et al.*, 1990, 1992; Reist *et al.*, 1989). One reason for the lack of clear evidence may be that the presence of psychiatric co-morbidity such as depression or generalized anxiety was not taken into account.

In terms of the therapists' response, the theory by Foa and colleagues linking various levels of disablement following events with differing associated threat is probably the most useful. The main aim of therapy derived from such a model should be to access all the fear structure held by the victim and to provide either contradictory information or to change the negative valence associated with the high arousal (anxious feelings) which occurs when elements in the fear structure are matched. This matching prompts behavioural and cognitive avoidance which prevents emotional processing (Rachman, 1980). It is the emotional processing which will reduce symptomatology.

THE NORMAL PROCESS OF RECOVERY

Following a serious assault, most victims experience a post-traumatic reaction, including recollections of the assault, rehearsing of preceding events, avoidance of features that recall the event and physiological hyperarousal. However, this brief and generally self-limiting reaction, which in most cases subsides within 4–6 weeks, is distinct from a full-blown post-traumatic stress disorder, which emphasizes a symptomatic period of 1 month's duration. There is still controversy about the precise factors that impede the appropriate cognitive processing of a trauma so that a post-traumatic 'reaction' develops into a post-traumatic stress disorder proper. Premorbid personality, the precise nature of the trauma and the quality of social support all make a contribution towards influencing the pattern and completeness of recovery after a traumatic event.

WHEN THERAPY IS REQUIRED

Various sorts of interventions can be provided for different levels of disablement and at different times following a violent incident. Not all victims will need one-to-one counselling but some acknowledgement of the impact of a violent incident is usually required by both victims and witnesses. Guidelines on the sorts of therapy that should be offered depending on the time since the incident and the severity of the reactions will now be discussed.

Debriefing

Initially, many people will experience post-traumatic reactions and it is thought that early intervention will prevent these from developing into anything more serious and will allow the therapists to identify those people who have been most seriously affected. The aim in this stage is to provide some reframing of the event so that it is understandable. Crisis theory (already discussed) offers a theoretical model on which to base such interventions. Such therapies that are based on this model are not well specified but they all include discussions with victims about the incident and a framing of psychological distress into normal responses to an abnormal incident.

Therapy for victims with severe disturbances

Different levels of disablement may require different layers of therapy. However, all involve accessing the fear structure, allowing some emotional processing and changing the beliefs incorporated into the fear structure. What follows is a discussion of the sorts of therapy required when symptoms are severe and interfere considerably with the victim's life.

The first issue in therapy is to access the fear structure and to allow some emotional processing to take place. The main difficulty for victims is the denial and avoidance of the event. This leads to avoidance of things that remind the person of the event but also the avoidance of the experience of emotions associated with the event. The following three types of interventions all encourage the subject to emotionally process the event either merely by allowing the victim to repeat it or by using other techniques.

Stress-inoculation training

This was developed by Meichenbaum (1985) and has subsequently been adapted to help victims of rape and sexual assault (Kilpatrick *et al.*, 1982). Treatment consists of two phases: the first is an education package in which the cognitive, emotional, physical and behavioural responses to fear are explained within a framework that is understandable and that makes sense to the victim. In the second phase, specific skills are taught to cope with target fears and their physical, behavioural and cognitive expressions. Skills taught for coping with fear in the physical channel are muscle relaxation and breathing control. Skills taught to deal with fear expressed through the behavioural channel are covert modelling and role playing and for the cognitive channel, thought stoppage and guided self-dialogue are used. Throughout this process the victim is encouraged to assess the actual probability of the feared event happening again, to manage the overwhelming fear and avoidance behaviour, to control self-criticism and self-devaluation and to engage in the feared behaviour. Throughout the process the victim is encouraged to carry out assignments to reinforce the learning process and homework in between sessions. The whole process generally lasts about 12 sessions (Calhoun and Atkeson, 1991, p. 70).

Disclosure

There is now some supporting evidence that the disclosure of upsetting or traumatic events can result in the reduction of stress-related illness (Pennebaker *et al.*, 1988). Routinely seeing individuals who have been assaulted in the course of their work and providing them with an opportunity to ventilate their feelings about what has happened may be not only appreciated by the victim but may also be extremely cost-effective for the organization in terms of diminishing stress-related illness and sick leave paid by the organization.

Imaginal exposure

More recently, activation of fear structures has been successfully carried out by using a technique of prolonged imaginal exposure to the event. Several reports of this sort of therapy are now in the literature and have shown extremely good results (Richards and Rose, 1991). Victims of traumas are asked to talk about the incident as if it were currently happening. The victim is also asked to include references to how they felt as they make their description. The first-person account produced in this way is recorded on a tape. The victims are then asked to listen to the tape several times as homework assignments. Further recordings are made in later sessions and often these recordings produce more detailed accounts, which suggests that the victim is now able to access more of the fear model. It also allows the victim to feel that they have more control over the memory of the incident. Dramatic reductions in symptoms have been shown over as few as two sessions.

Other treatment objectives are to cut down the number of uncontrolled exposures to stimuli that provoke fear. This can be carried out by requiring the victim to expose themselves following a specific hierarchy. For instance, a victim who has developed a phobia of a place may have to be introduced back into the environment slowly. This element of therapy is based on strict behavioural principles.

It is also important to investigate the person's appraisal of elements of the event. How dangerous was the event in objective terms and does this differ from the victim's perception? Are the victim's perceptions of the event extremely negative? Is there anything positive that the victim has learned from the experience? This element of therapy is based on cognitive behavioural principles.

TREATMENT ISSUES FOR VICTIMS OF VIOLENCE AT WORK

Professional versus informal counselling and support

The victim should be allowed a choice of professional or informal counselling that does not lead to further victimization. There are some advantages to providing professional counselling. First, there is a clearly defined structural relationship from a professional rather than a volunteer in which it may be safer to explore painful issues. Second, there may be closer matching of treatment to difficulties. The treatment of the reactions to traumatic events can bring into consciousness other events in the past, such as a previous death that still evokes painful memories or other victim experiences. A trained professional counsellor would be able to deal with these recollections as they arise and reduce their painful consequences.

Confidentiality

There has been a dispute running through the literature on treatment of whether counselling should be provided in a confidential relationship or whether some of the information should be available to the employer. Nevertheless, even those who suggest limited confidentiality do not agree on why and what sort of information would be relevant to an employer. Professional organizations such as the British Association of Social Workers (BASW, 1988) concluded that counselling relationships may reveal information on serious disciplinary or criminal offences committed by colleagues that may have led directly to the incident. The victim should be encouraged to report these offences themselves and, as a last resort, they might be reported by the counsellor to the appropriate authorities. Others who are more closely allied to employers' organizations (White and Hatcher, 1988) would like information to be provided to the employer to affect the managerial decisions pertinent to the future job demands on the employee victim. The emphasis throughout this book has been on treating the victims of violence at work in the same way as any other victim. In our view, they should receive medical and psychological care like any other victim – confidential, objective and impartial care given away from the work unit.

Treatment within or separate from the organization

The separateness of the support provided is related to confidentiality in that many staff feel that any support provided from within the organization is subject to different rules than therapeutic relationships, which are structurally separate. Certainly support that is only designed to be provided from line managers may be inappropriate, as any information divulged could be perceived as having implications for the person's future career. It has been suggested that occupational health units may be able to provide such a service as they can provide expertise and have less associated stigma.

Normalizing symptoms

Victims need to be assured that fear symptoms (e.g. pounding heart, trembling body) are characteristics of hyperarousal and are normal following the incident. The person is likely to become more irritable and find that small incidents provoke extreme reactions. They may also experience nightmares involving recreation of the event and often dreams of helplessness increase. It is important to emphasize that all these symptoms are normal reactions to an abnormal event.

Anger

Anger may be displaced onto others and even when offers of support are made they may produce an initial outburst. Sometimes victims may not be able to cope with these strong emotions and will therefore push supporters away. Significant others may also need professional help to maintain their supportive stance.

MODELS OF SUPPORT ALREADY PROVIDED

There are several different models of intervention that have been provided to health care staff – most are centred on hospitals but they all have common elements that could be combined in different ways for different groups of health professionals without such a clearly defined geographical base. Table 11.1 provides an overview of the sorts of interventions that have been suggested or tried. Most have not been running for long enough to provide a clear evaluation and there have been no comparative studies to investigate the acceptability of the different schemes for staff. Schemes also involve different numbers of elements and therefore have quite different cost implications for an organization. These costs have not yet been quantified, especially in relation to the observed benefits.

Table 11.1 Models of support

Element of intervention	Flannery et al. (1991)	Morrison (1988)	Engel and Marsh (1986)	Dawson et al. (1988)
Specific support team	x			x
24 h cover (telephone at night?)	x			?
Crisis intervention:				
Immediate assessment for being sent home	x	x		?
Debriefing	x			?
Ensuring not alone at home	x			?
Counselling/support	x	x	x	x
Group work with victims	x			?
Access to private counselling	x	x	x	
Time off for any of the above activities	x			?
Debriefing for other staff not directly involved	x	x		?
Possible family meetings for staff	x			?
Further contact at set intervals	x	x		?

One of the main differences among the models is the employment of a specific team of individuals whose sole duty is to provide post-violence support. Flannery *et al.* (1991) describe the most comprehensive service. Their assault team provides a 24 hour service for debriefing staff, making assessments of injuries and the victim's current social supports. Their emphasis is on initial debriefing followed by a comprehensive system of support through further contacts, work in groups, support for families and help for other staff not directly involved in the incident. Some staff may be offered professional counselling outside this context but this is expected to be rare. Other services also stress the need for comprehensive cover and the need for initial support. In fact, some emphasize the need for support rather than counselling during the initial contacts, although usually the victim can have access to professional counselling if they wish.

Other schemes provide less comprehensive care. Some provide only debriefing through managerial staff, for example clinical nurse managers who are designated to provide this service on a rota or via a buddy system. One example is provided by Morrison (1988) who suggests strict time periods within which staff and victims should be seen by ward staff. The managers in this service provide a monitoring service and it is their responsibility to provide a follow-up interview with the victim 6–8 weeks after the incident. Day-to-day support is expected to be provided by colleagues and there is no obvious link with external counsellors. In the buddy system (Dawson *et al.*, 1988), the Assault Support Team is contacted and the particular person on duty then contacts the victim and 'depending on the needs of the victim' will see them immediately or schedule a meeting in the near future. Engel and Marsh (1986) provide a self-referral counselling service, which is offered to staff following an incident. However, this is not a comprehensive service and it is not clear what sort of counselling is provided or for how long.

HELP FROM OUTSIDE THE ORGANIZATION

Occasionally it may be helpful to seek assistance from external agencies or individuals who are not themselves connected with the organization. Victims of assault may be reluctant to seek help from colleagues or to acknowledge that they are having difficulty in recovering from their victimization. The hierarchical structure within the NHS means that nursing staff and professionals in training grades who are most at risk of assault are dependent on their managers to provide them with references and ensure their progression up the professional ladder. Professional competence may appear to be incompatible with prolonged feelings of vulnerability and distress following a violent incident at work and may therefore make victims reluctant to seek help from their colleagues and managers. Equally, there is considerable resistance against the medicalization or 'psychiatrization' of problems experienced by individuals who see themselves as carers rather than being cared for. While several individuals may derive support and make sense of their assaults through discussions with family members, friends and within a social network outside the work environment, there are some individuals who have no access to a supportive social network or who feel that close friends would be unable to provide a dispassionate and sufficiently emotionally detached response to their distress. It is therefore crucial that all individuals within the Health Service are provided with alternative avenues of help.

Victims of assault in the workplace experience similar problems to victims of crime in the community. The National Association of Victim Support schemes offer assistance to victims of crime at several levels. First, the volunteers provide information in relation to the anticipated responses to the crime, the duration and likely pattern of those responses, the processing of complaints within the criminal justice system including the mechanism of receiving compensation, assisting in a victim's immediate practical needs, for example transporting the individual to and from the police stations, accompanying them to out-patient clinics, assisting in re-housing etc. (Reeves, 1985). Alongside these functions the Victim Support scheme volunteers offer support for the victims of crime along the model of crisis intervention (Caplan, 1964) to facilitate their emotional recovery.

While there is no particular political ideology underlying the growth of victim-support schemes they emphasize the fact that workers operate on a volunteer basis, without pay, thus removing concerns about the medicalization of essential normal responses and additionally operate a practice of outreach whereby volunteers visit victims in their own home. The frequency of these visits is determined by the individual's level of distress and thus provides a more immediate and individually tailored response to victimization than professional organizations would practically be able to offer (MaGuire, 1985).

Victim-support schemes accept most referrals from the police but direct self-referral is becoming an increasingly accepted part of the scheme's workload and victims of violence in the workplace may find that the intervention of a dispassionate but 'empathic' and informed third party who does not seek to blame or find explanations for what has happened is reassuring. There are several government documents that are enthusiastic about this means of support for victims at work (Health Services Advisory Committee, 1987) and recent empirical studies have shown that when support is available it is highly valued by victims (e.g. Whittington and Wykes, 1992).

A MODEL FOR INTERVENTION

In general, anyone who approaches the victim must provide unquali-fied, empathic support and be acutely aware of not appearing to attribute any blame to the victim. Qualified support and counselling are necessary and, in some cases, may be essential but informal peer support is also effective in reducing the consequences of an incident.

Immediate needs of victims

The most immediate needs will have to be dealt with by personnel within the organization and so there is a need to train them to be able to respond appropriately. Issues of training are discussed in Chapter 12.

Safety and physical reassurance

In the immediate aftermath of an incident, the victim's primary need is to feel safe. The victim should not be ignored or left alone. He or she should be removed from the place where the incident occurred as soon as it is safe to do so. If it is not possible to take victims out of the environment entirely then they should at least be offered some respite and time-out from the situation, for example, by having a cup of tea. If there are several victims, then those who are overwrought, crying, etc. should be dealt with first. It may not be helpful to stop people from working if they wish to. Victims may want to ensure that they still can function.

There is also a need to help with immediate problem-solving in order to decide about the future safety and protection of the victim and other staff. This requires specific information from the victim about the details of the incident and therefore an initial debriefing of the victim is important. The victim must be assessed by a competent source to evaluate the extent of injuries and the need for treatment. This should be carried out by an occupational health service, the victim's own GP or the local casualty department. The victim may need to be provided with immediate transportation in order to be assessed. It should also be the responsibility of the organization to ensure that the victim is not alone at home for a short period after the incident. Apart from the safety issues, victims have a need for pastoral care and the support provided by colleagues, family and friends is very important in the immediate aftermath. One person from the work environment should assume responsibility for keeping in touch with the victim during any absence.

Immediate debriefing

This is so that each person can pass on relevant information and express their feelings about the event. It is possible that this intervention alone will help the person to structure his or her thoughts about the incident and put it into perspective. The immediate provision of support also indicates a recognition from the organization that a significant event has taken place.

The immediate care of the victim will rely mainly on colleagues but it is useful to have an external agency providing all staff with support. Large organizations, such as hospitals or social services, should be able to provide suitable trained staff from within the organization who can react quickly to any incident. Smaller organizations, such as health centres, may be able to join with others to buy in such a service from suitably qualified staff, or may wish to designate certain staff for specific training in this area. The specific elements of a postincident support package will be dependent on the level of suspected risk and the cost of different models.

Medium-term interventions

Staff who have more serious psychological difficulties should be provided with the opportunity for further counselling from trained personnel, either within or external to the agency but, in either case, respecting the confidentiality of both the contact and the information divulged. Counselling should take the form of a structure to reduce behavioural, emotional and cognitive avoidance, while increasing coping and competency skills. The use of imaginal desensitization (Richards and Rose, 1991) seems to provide a tool that has proven to be cost-effective, together with the provision of some desensitization, to both the people and events, that leads to re-experiencing of the event.

Longer-term interventions

Apart from training in the skills required to prevent violence, management of violence training should also include the provision of information about the short-term and possibly longer-term consequences of being involved in a violent incident. This knowledge may then allow members of the caring professions to acknowledge their own feelings and prevent some of the more serious psychological sequelae. Not all violence can be prevented and it is therefore important for the caring professions to acknowledge that, although they have many social and professional skills, unpredictable and uncontrollable events will occur. This acknowledgement may reduce self-blame and should certainly reduce the victimization by colleagues.

Several possible interventions within the workplace that could reduce the psychological effects of violent incidents have been suggested in this chapter. Helping an individual has the immediate benefit to an organization by aiding their return to work and using their skills in the workplace. It also has an effect on the whole workforce. By officially recognizing the problems, the morale of the workforce will increase; this has effects on all aspects of productivity and quality of service.

REFERENCES

American Psychiatric Association (1987) *Diagnostic and Statistical Manual of Mental Disorders*, revised 3rd edn, APA, Washington DC.

BASW (1988) *Violence to Social Workers*, British Association of Social Workers, Birmingham.

Brodsky, S. (1976) Rape at work, in *Sexual Assault: The Victim and the Rapist*, (eds M. Walker and S. Brodsky), Lexington, Lexington, Massachusetts.

Calhoun, K.S. and Atkeson, B.M. (1991) *Treatment of Rape Victims: Facilitating Psychosocial Adjustment*, Pergamon Press, Oxford.

Caplan (1964) *Principles of Preventive Psychiatry*, Basic Books, New York.

Davidson, J. (1992) Drug therapy of post-traumatic stress disorder. *British Journal of Psychiatry*, **160**, 309–15.

Davidson, J., Kudler, H., Smith, R. *et al.* (1990) Treatment of post-traumatic stress disorder with amitryptiline and placebo. *Archives of General Psychiatry*, **47**, 259–66.

Davidson, J., Kudler, H. and Smith, R. (1992) Assessment and pharmacotherapy of post-traumatic stress disorder, in *Biological Assessment and Treatment of Post-Traumatic Stress Disorder*, (ed. E.L. Giller), APP, Washington.

Dawson, J., Johnson, M., Kehiayan, N. *et al.* (1988) Response to patient assault: A peer-support programme for nurses. *Journal of Psychosocial Nursing and Mental Health Services*, **26**(2), 8–15.

Engel, F. and Marsh, S. (1986) Helping the employee victim of violence in hospitals, *Hospital and Community Psychiatry*, **37**, 159–62.

Foa, E. and Kozak, M. (1986) Emotional processing of fear: Exposure to corrective information, *Psychological Bulletin*, **99**, 20–35.

Foa, E., Steketee, G. and Rothbaum, B. (1989) Behavioural/cognitive conceptualizations of post-traumatic stress disorder. *Behaviour Therapy*, **20**, 155–76.

Flannery, R.B., Fulton, P., Tausch, J. *et al.* (1991) A programme to help staff cope with the psychological sequelae of assaults by patients. *Hospital and Community Psychiatry*, **42**, 935–38.

Giller, E.L. (1990) *Biological Assessment and Treatment of Post-Traumatic Stress Disorder*. APS, Washington.

Health Services Advisory Committee (1987) *Violence to Staff in the Health Services*, Health and Safety Commission, London.

Kilpatrick, D.G., Veronon, L.J. and Resick, P.A. (1982) Psychological sequelae to rape: Assessment and treatment strategies, in *Behavioural Medicine: Assessment and Treatment Strategies*, (eds D.M. Dolays and R.L. Meredith), Plenum Press, New York.

Lindeman, E. (1944) Symptomatology in Management of Acute Grief. *American Journal of Psychiatry*, **101**, 141–48.

MaGuire, M. (1985) Victims' needs and victims' services: Indications from research. *Victimology: An International Journal*, **10**, 1–4, 539–59.

Meichenbaum, D.H. (1985) *Stress-inoculation training*, Pergamon Press, Elmsford, New York.

Mezey, G. and Rubenstein, M. (1992) Sexual harassment: the problem and its consequences. *Journal of Forensic Psychiatry*, **3**, 221–33.

Morrison, E. (1988) The assaulted nurse: Strategies for healing. *Perspectives in Psychiatric Care*, **24**, 120–26.

Mowrer, O.H. (1947) On the dual nature of learning: A reinterpretation of 'conditioning' and 'problem-solving'. *Harvard Educational Review*, **17**, 102–48.

Ochberg, F. (1988) *Post-Traumatic Therapy and the Victims of Violence*, Brunner/Mazel, New York.

Parkes, C.M. (1975) *Bereavement: Studies of Grief in Adult Life*. Penguin, London.

Pennebaker, J.W., Kiecolt-Glaser, J.K., Glaser, J.K. *et al.* (1988) Disclosure of traumas and immune function: Health implications for psychotherapy. *Journal of Consulting and Clinical Psychology*, **56**(2), 239–45.

Rachman, S.J. (1980) Emotional processing. *Behavior Research and Therapy*, **18**, 51–60.

Reeves, H. (1985) Victims' support schemes: The United Kingdom model. *Victimology: An International Journal*, **10**, 679–86.

Reist, C., Kauffman, C., Haier, R. *et al.* (1989) A controlled trial of desiprimine in 18 men with post-traumatic stress disorder. *American Journal of Psychiatry*, **146**, 513–16.

Richards, D. and Rose, J. (1991) Exposure therapy for post-traumatic stress disorder. *British Journal of Psychiatry*, **158**, 836–40.

Silverman, D.C. (1978) Sharing the crisis of rape: Counselling the mates and families of victims. *American Journal of Ortho Psychiatry*, **48**, 166–73.

Van der Kolk, B.A. (1987) The drug treatment of post-traumatic stress disorder. *Journal of Affective Disorders*, **13**, 203–13.

Van der Kolk, B.A., Greenberg, M., Boyd, H. *et al.* (1985) Inescapable shock, neurotransmitters and addiction to trauma, towards a psychobiology of post-traumatic stress. *Biological Psychiatry*, **20**, 314–25.

White, S. and Hatcher, C. (1988) Violence and the trauma response. *Occupational Medicine State-of-the-Art Reviews*, **3**(4).

Whittington, R. and Wykes, T. (1992) Staff strain and social support in a psychiatric hospital following assault by a patient. *Journal of Advanced Nursing*, **17**, 480–86.

CHAPTER 12

Organizational approaches to the prevention and management of violence

Anne Greaves

INTRODUCTION

Violence is the most life-threatening risk faced by health care staff at work. Surveys show how commonplace it is and, as well as the risk of injury, it can bring unmanageable levels of occupational stress that damage the staff's personal esteem and threaten their ability to continue in the job.

Violence at work is not something that has to be accepted as part of a contract of employment. It cannot just be dismissed as 'bad luck', incompetence or the result of individual personalities. Neither is it just a law-and-order issue. The use of the word 'crime' in describing violence at work is unhelpful and it prevents a proper examination of the underlying causes and changes needed to combat it.

The risk of violence is work-related. It arises directly out of the jobs people are asked to do and the circumstances in which they have to work. This is shown diagrammatically in Figure 12.1. Despite being an organizational issue, violence at work appears to be one of the work-related risks that employees are expected to cope with alone. They are expected to use their experience and professional training to identify when they are at risk and then to determine how they can cope with that risk. Much of the risk of violence in the health care sector is predictable (i.e. foreseeable) and therefore preventable if tackled in a systematic way by the organization. Many employers have handed their responsibility for managing this health and safety problem to their employees. Focusing only on the employee is unlikely to provide a solution because this ignores the multitude of other factors involved.

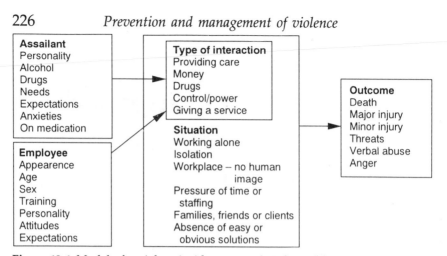

Figure 12.1 Model of a violent incident at work (adapted from *Violence to Staff – A Basis for Assessment and Prevention*, HSE, 1989).

THE LEGAL POSITION

Employers, or more specifically their representatives in management, have a duty of care for the health and safety of their employees and, in relation to the risk of violence, this duty is also a statutory one. Under the Health and Safety at Work Act 1974, employers have a duty to provide for the health and safety of their employees and this covers those employees who face a foreseeable (predictable) risk of violence.

For too long this responsibility has been ignored or minimized, despite the fact that some health care staff have been killed, others have suffered injury and many face a daily dose of violence at work. To understand the employers' reluctance to manage effectively this aspect of their health and safety responsibilities, it is necessary to look at the nature of the legal responsibilities placed on employers by health and safety legislation.

The main responsibility of employers is set out in section 2 of the Act: 'It shall be the duty of every employer to ensure, so far as is reasonably practicable, the health, safety and welfare at work of all his employees'. The report of the DHSS Committee on Violence set up under Lord Skelmersdale after the death of a social worker in 1986 stated that: 'Where violent incidents are foreseeable employers have a duty under section 2 of that Act to identify the nature and extent of the risk and to devise measures which provide a safe workplace and a safe system of work'.

The Health and Safety at Work Act 1974 was a major innovation in UK health and safety law. Its introduction meant that health and safety law applied to all employers, all workplaces and all risks. However, the duties it places on employers are set down in very general terms, as aims to be achieved. By implication, it requires employers to look at the nature of their own organizations and ask questions about whether anything about the workplace or the work activity could pose a risk to the health and safety of employees. If so then the employer is required to introduce measures to remove or control the identified risks.

From 1 January 1993, the Management of Health and Safety at Work Regulations were introduced in the UK to comply with the European Framework Directive. They place new duties on employers and make explicit the duties of employers already set out in the Health and Safety at Work Act 1974. However, they also embody the European approach to the management of health and safety at work where the emphasis is placed on risk assessment. This is the removal of risk at source and the introduction of comprehensive, preventative strategies to control those risks that cannot be eliminated. The key phrases for any manager in the health care sector are 'risk assessment' and 'coherent overall preventative policy'. Such a policy should cover technology, organization of work, working conditions, social relationships and the influence of factors relating to the working environment. Piecemeal arrangements made in response to an incident will no longer be sufficient.

THE RESPONSE OF EMPLOYERS

The legal context has had an enormous effect on employers' attitudes to their responsibility in health and safety. The Health and Safety at Work Act 1974 introduced a concept of a systematic approach to the management of health and safety within an organization. For the first time UK law did not tell employers what the risks to health and safety were and what to do to remain lawful. This revolutionary change bemused many employers and gave some the opportunity to use the general wording of the Act to argue that it did not apply to many of the specific situations that arose in work and so required no action from them.

Pre-1974 legislation

Some of this employer resistance can only be understood by appreciating the change in the concept of health and safety management that the Health and Safety at Work Act 1974 brought. Until then, the UK law only applied to precisely defined workplaces and only covered specific hazards, leaving the impression that anything that was excluded from the legislation presented no problems and therefore needed no action. Employers wishing to meet their legal responsibilities had first to decide if their premises fitted the precise definitions of a factory, building operation, office, shop or railway premises, etc.

If not, then there was no statutory responsibility to provide for the health and safety of employees, only the duty of care under common law. If the premises did match the definition then all the employer had to do was to look at what the Act or Regulation contained and respond. However, this would not mean that the employer, although meeting the legal obligations set out in statute law, was providing for the health and safety of employees. This is because the pre-1974 legislation often ignored known hazards; for example, it would require that employees were protected from the moving parts of machinery but not from the harmful noise levels the machinery could produce or from the oil that it could spray onto the skin of employees.

The pre-1974 UK legislation on health and safety delivered another message to the health care sector that has been unhelpful and long-standing. UK law was originally developed to meet the health and safety problems created in the manufacturing sector. This historical inheritance created a mythology that work outside of manufacturing and construction does not bring health and safety problems and is safe, healthy and comfortable. This mythology is so ingrained that it remains despite the HSW Act which introduced statutory responsibilities to the whole of the health care sector. Employers in the health care sector more easily accepted the need to introduce preventative measures for the use of radiation and harmful substances but not other hazards such as violence.

This led to an approach to the management of health and safety that was mechanistic and ill-suited to cope with some of the more complex work-related health problems that occur in the workplace. It fostered a concept of a single cause and a single solution for health and safety problems. It did not prepare employers for the requirements of the approach embodied in the HSW Act.

The effects post-1974

After 1974 employers could no longer turn to the statute to discover what they must do to remain lawful. Instead they found that they had to become involved in systematic risk assessment and to take responsibility for the health and safety problems created by the nature of their organization. It also meant that they had to recognize the whole range of health and safety problems facing their employees.

European initiatives on health and safety will force a change on those managers in the health care sector who, to date, have given little priority to the management of health and safety or ignored authoritative advice. Decisions about priorities for legislation on health and safety are now made in Europe with member states being required to introduce legislation to meet any Directives adopted by the European Council of Ministers. The European emphasis is on a coherent overall preventative strategy based on risk assessment carried out by competent persons. It stresses the need for information and training for employees and consultation with trade union safety representatives.

DEFINING VIOLENCE AT WORK

This is an essential, if difficult, first step for anyone involved in the investigation, management and prevention of violence at work. It is not sufficient to limit the definition to violence leading to injury. Violent incidents were classified by the Health and Safety Commission Health Services Advisory Committee (HSC/HSAC), in its guidance published in 1987, as those leading to (i) death; (ii) major injury (requiring medical assistance); (iii) minor injury (requiring only first aid); (iv) threats with weapons or implements even if no physical injury occurs, and (v) verbal abuse.

The report of the DHSS Committee also chose a wider definition:

> The application of force, severe threat or serious abuse, by members of the public towards people arising out of their work whether or not they are on duty; and it includes severe verbal abuse or threat where this is judged likely to turn into actual violence; serious harassment (including racial or sexual harassment); threat with a weapon; major or minor injury; fatality.
>
> *(DHSS, 1988)*

However, violent incidents are not limited to the workplace and can take place anywhere in the community and at the home of the worker. Nevertheless, the violence still counts as work-related as it arises out of the course of employment. The definition in the Health and Safety Executive's (1989) free booklet *Violence to Staff* recognizes this aspect of violence at work. It defines violence at work as: 'Any incident in which an employee is exposed, threatened or assaulted by a member of the public in circumstances arising out of the course of his or her employment'.

A COMMITMENT TO PREVENTION

It is in the interests of management to acknowledge the risk to employees and to make a commitment to develop policies to prevent the predictable violence. This is not only because health and safety law requires this but because of the costs of failing to do anything. The risk of violence can increase absenteeism because staff are hurt and afraid. Some may leave and so the investment in training inexperienced staff will be lost. There could be litigation, bad publicity and certainly low morale among staff, all very costly to the employer in the long term. It is even more important in the health care sector where managements rely heavily on the commitment and contribution of a stable, experienced workforce.

Employers need to make a public statement to the staff that all violence to staff is unacceptable and, whatever the reason for it, will not be seen as a failing on the part of a member of staff or be seen as a required part of any job. One large local authority prefaced its policy document for residential work with the following statement:

> ... Council fully accepts the responsibility to endeavour to reduce risks to staff by introducing preventative and protective measures, by issuing clear policies and procedures and by developing the ability of employees to manage and deal with violent incidents. In giving such commitment to developing the department's capacity to control and handle violence the Council also acknowledges that, in most cases, involvement in violent incidents should not reflect adversely on staff concerned or be viewed as poor practice.

If managements continue to fail to take this issue seriously they will lose the goodwill of their staff and workers and their unions could respond in a traditional way. Strathclyde created its policy after residential workers had been on strike about violence at work. Senior psychiatric social workers in Manchester refused to do home visits in a particular area until the risk of violence to them was treated seriously. Psychiatrists also refused to carry out domiciliary visits in one part of their inner city district. All these staff responses have resulted in policy changes, some on a local basis and others (on trainee psychiatrists) on a national basis. However, this level of staff response would not be necessary if employers developed their own policies.

THE NEED FOR PROCEDURES

It is important that management do not adopt the philosophy that they alone can develop a policy on the management and prevention of violence. The Management of Health and Safety at Work Regulations require employers from 1 January 1993 to involve workers and their representatives in decisions about the assessment of risk and the measures to be taken to eliminate or control that risk. In the UK, this will mean the involvement of trade union safety representatives. Staff are an invaluable information resource and they will work better if they feel that they have been party to decisions about the workplace and working practices. Their trade unions provide arrangements whereby management can involve workers.

THE AIMS OF ANY POLICY

The overall aim is obviously the prevention of injuries and damage to the health of staff. The employers' commitment will, however, have to be delineated more precisely than this. The policy will need to outline the actions the employer is prepared to make to achieve safe workplaces and safe working methods for staff. It should include details of the methods of risk-assessment and for monitoring the effectiveness of preventative measures. It will need to define the system for reporting and recording incidents and the support available to staff who have been exposed to violence. It should make clear the responsibilities of managers and supervisors and what employees should do if an incident occurs. It should also cover the training implications.

This should not appear as a daunting task for management. It is simply the application of systematic management techniques to a health and safety problem, which is serious for the health care sector. It is not dissimilar to the action required from employers to comply with the Control of Substances Hazardous to Health Regulations 1990 (COSHH). Authoritative advice from the HSE (1989), HSAC (1987), the DHSS Committee on Violence (1988) and the Association of Directors of Social Services (1987) has been published, more advice on the issue of violence at work than was available when the COSHH Regulations became law on 1 January 1990. Notwithstanding, management felt able to tackle COSHH but still appear reluctant to deal with the risk of violence.

Current legislation indicates that a systematic approach to any health and safety issue involves at least three main stages:

1. Risk-assessment;
2. Introduction of preventative measures; and
3. Monitoring.

These are outlined later in this chapter.

There are a variety of ways of achieving a policy. The important thing is that it should be systematic, involve workers and set itself clear objectives. When Strathclyde Regional Council decided to look at the need to reduce the level of violence in residential homes a Working Party was set up, including management, trade union representatives and members of staff who worked in the residential sector. The Working Party set itself tasks and commissioned a literature search as well as seeking information from other local authorities. The report of the Working Party set several objectives for the achievement of change: (i) immediate (within the next 12 months); (ii) intermediate (for resolution now and action within 2–5 years); and (iii) long-term (for action within 5–10 years). This is a useful model for all those setting up a policy.

It is important that employers are clear about what is involved in developing strategies to prevent violence to staff. For some employers acknowledging that the problem exists induces a sense of impotence; they search for a 'blueprint' – a step by step guide on what to do – or they resort to a single solution that they believe will deal with the problem. Blueprints and panaceas do not exist but guidance and experience of facing violence do.

The DHSS report (DHSS, 1988) made it very clear that all managers should take every threat of violence seriously. The report also stated that central strategies alone would be insufficient since they must take account of specific local circumstances. This means that each job must be investigated separately and may need its own specific preventative measures. These local strategies must also include procedures for the management of violent situations and for the counselling and support of staff who have faced violence. The report clearly states that trade unions have a role in the devising of such a strategy at local level.

When launching the HSE document, Dr John Cullen (now Sir John Cullen), then Chair of the Health and Safety Commission, said:

> The report makes clear that the way jobs are planned and performed can affect the occurrence of violence. It emphasises the importance of a systematic approach to the design and monitoring of preventative measures. It should help employers who are uncertain about the extent of violence to their staff as

1. Do staff in your unit/district have contact with the public during which violence may occur?
   (Yes = 1; No = 0) □

2. Does a violence problem exist?
   (Yes = 1; Don't know = 1; No = 0) □

3. If you are unsure, are you finding out more by taking soundings from managers and staff?
   (Yes = 0; No = 1) □

4. If there is known to be a problem, do you have a proper system for recording assaults, in sufficient detail?
   (Yes = 0; No = 1) □

5. Do you regularly analyse the data as a basis for deciding what measures may be needed?
   (Yes = 0; No = 1) □

6. Have suitable prevention measures been adopted?
   (Yes = 0; No = 1) □

7. Is the problem and your general approach to dealing with it referred to in your written safety policy?
   (Yes = 0; No = 1) □

8. (i) Have previous measures proved effective and (ii) is their effectiveness monitored?
   (Yes to both = 0; No to either (i) or (ii) = 1) □

Figure 12.2 Checklist for assessing the risk of violence to be used by managers in consultation with staff.

well as those who recognize the problem but are unsure of how best to devise effective measures to combat it.

The simple checklist shown in Figure 12.2 is adapted from the HSAC guidance for managers who are just beginning to plan how to tackle the risk of violence. If there are any scores of 1 or more a specific review of policies or their development is necessary.

RISK ASSESSMENT

Employers have a duty to make an assessment of the risks to the health and safety of their employees. This need not be a complex process but it must be systematic if it is to achieve its aims. The purpose of carrying out a risk assessment is to identify:

- the extent and nature of the risk;
- the factors that contribute to the risk, the causes; and
- changes necessary to eliminate or control the risk.

If there are five or more employees the Management of Health and Safety at Work Regulations require, from 1 January 1993, that this assessment must be written down and regularly revised. It would be good management practice to record the assessment anyway so that it becomes a resource in planning the preventative measures and at the monitoring stage.

RECORDED INCIDENTS

A first step would be to look in detail at the incidents that have already occurred. While an obvious starting point, this probably highlights one of the first problems that face many managers when they begin to deal with work-related violence. Many violent incidents are not reported or recorded in a systematic way.

Clearly a systematic method of recording violent incidents is essential but it will only work if staff are willing to report incidents. Therefore it is important to consider carefully the reasons why staff have in the past been reluctant to report incidents. Staff will not report incidents unless they are confident about the reception such a report will receive from management and that it will lead to some action, some changes to bring about a reduction in the risk of violence in the future.

Many staff have the fear, and some the experience, that involvement in a violent incident will be seen as their failure; their mishandling of a situation and be regarded as professional incompetence. Some are already so distressed by the experience that they do not want the attention a report will bring. With no access to counselling and support they see no point in adding to their own distress.

A reporting system will only work if it is one part of an overall strategy that can be seen to be tackling this serious work-related risk. When establishing a recording system, management must decide what information they need; why they need the information and how they intend to use it.

One question of concern to everyone at work is whether or not the incidence of violence to staff has increased. Without proper records it is impossible to answer this question. Violent incidents at work have been seen as different from other accidents at work and so managements have not included them in their accident-recording systems. The regulations that require employers to record accidents, dangerous occurrences and occupational ill health (The Reporting of Injuries, Diseases and Dangerous Occurrences Regulations 1985) are being revised and it is believed that violent incidents will be made reportable.

No employer or manager should assume that because they are not aware of any violent incidents to their staff, they do not have a problem to manage. As the HSE found, an incident in one organization was regarded as isolated until soundings were made and it was found that violence was much more common and affected a wider range of jobs than first thought. Even when a work-related fatality from violence occurs the usual shocked response is to describe it as a one-off, something totally unexpected that could not be avoided. Yet investigations of these deaths produce reports of other injuries, and threats and circumstances that indicate the existence of predictable risk.

In the NHS there is, however, more than anecdotal evidence on the extent of violence to staff. When the HSAC was preparing its guidance for the health service, a large and serious survey was undertaken by the HSE on the level of violence reported by staff in a representative sample of health authorities (Chapter 1 for details).

The survey showed that in the previous 12 months:

- one in 200 (0.5%) staff had reported violence leading to major injury;
- more than 1 in 10 (11%) reported minor injuries needing first aid;
- 1 in 21 (4.6%) had been threatened with weapons and implements; and
- more than 1 in 6 (17.5%) had been threatened verbally.

The survey also found that the incidents of violence were not limited to any specific groups of staff but occurred across the whole range of NHS occupations.

While accepting the need for proper reporting of violent incidents leading to injuries, there is often some scepticism about the need to record threats if verbal abuse and no injury occurs. However, there is no need to assume that all types of violence should be recorded in the same way. The basic questions are why is the information needed and what will be done with it. In at least two of the work-related fatalities, the assailant issued a threat well in advance of the killing. It could make sense to have a different system for reporting and recording threats – a system that triggers the need for immediate action to support the member of staff and bring in assistance to watch for the assailant.

Verbal abuse should not be disregarded just because it is common, but clearly staff are unlikely to want to fill in a report form each time it occurs. However, verbal abuse may lead to physical violence and contributes dramatically to the level of stress experienced by staff. If there are regular staff meetings then it should be a standing item on the agenda, so long as there is discussion about causes and how things could be changed. Staff could be given a diary sheet where they indicate by ticking under a series of headings their perception of the level of verbal abuse each working period. However, these records will have to be discussed with staff or they will be seen as a token paper exercise.

INVESTIGATING THE POTENTIAL FOR RISK

Counting those who have already been damaged is only one way to assess the level of risk. By then staff have already been hurt physically and psychologically. The second approach is to follow the philosophy set out in the Health and Safety at Work Act 1974 and the Management of Health and Safety at Work Regulations, which is to question if there is anything about the jobs staff are asked to do, how these jobs are done and the circumstances in which staff work that could place them at risk from violence. This recognizes that it is not necessary to wait for incidents to occur before identifying the potential for risk or the risk that is inherent in some jobs. For the assessment to be suitable and sufficient it must indicate the causal factors so that it leads to preventative and protective measures that will be effective. The HSE booklet provides a list of risk factors:

- handling money or valuables;
- providing care, advice or training;
- carrying out inspection or enforcement duties;
- working with mentally disturbed, drunk or potentially violent people; or
- working alone.

By looking at the jobs people do and the context in which they work in the health care sector it is possible to identify the potential for violence.

RISK FACTORS

Jobs

In the health care sector there are jobs that require staff to:

- handle money;
- handle drugs or have access to them;
- provide care to people who are ill, distressed, afraid, in a panic and on medication;
- relate to people who have a great deal of anger, resentment and feelings of failure;
- meet people's unrealistically high expectations of what staff have to offer and their search for quick and easy solutions to very complex problems;
- face the friends and families of clients who may also be concerned, anxious, afraid and feel inadequate in relation to the large organization from which they are seeking help;
- work with people who have always used violence to express themselves or to achieve their needs; and
- exercise power to restrict the freedom of individuals to do exactly as they wish, e.g. power to recommend that children should not be left with a family; hospitalize others or to release others into the community whether they wish that to happen or not.

The circumstances in which jobs are performed

Some jobs are undertaken in such a way that health care staff:

- work in isolation from colleagues and other members of the public;
- work in clients' homes, in units that are physically isolated, and at hours when few other staff are around;
- have to follow procedures that provide little information to clients about what is happening;
- work in units that do not have a human image – these are often crowded, busy and lacking in some essentials for the public (e.g. access to refreshments, the telephone and toys for children); and
- work under pressures created by increased workloads, staff shortages and the absence of alternative support that can be offered to the client.

For the purpose of making a proper risk assessment it is essential to separate out individual causes of risk but it is equally important to recognize that these causes rarely appear in isolation. More often staff face a series of risk factors in any one situation – such as working with anxious, sick clients in isolation from colleagues (as shown in Figure 12.3).

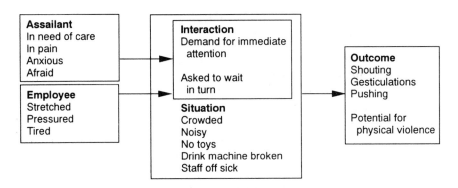

Figure 12.3 An incident in the health care sector (adapted from *Violence to Staff – A Basis for Assessment and Prevention*, HSE, 1989).

It is also important to recognize that work does not take place in isolation from society and attitudes and pressures that are created outside of the work situation will be brought into the workplace and can add to the risk of violence. Racism and sexism will influence the way staff are treated by the public and the way the people can be treated by the staff. Equally, the common belief that those working in the public sector are less efficient and have an easier ride compared with those in the private sector will affect attitudes and expectations of clients.

In addition, changes in society can increase the pressure on those working in the health care sector. Clients may feel they have waited too long for help or see the health care worker as their last chance to get help. It could also mean that by the time some people appear they are desperate, having not received help because other agencies have disappeared or are overstretched. Changes in management structures and style and the level of resources available increase the pressure. While managers in the health care sector may feel they have no responsibility for these external factors, it would be remiss to ignore their influence when determining risk or in influencing the effectiveness of any preventative measures.

PREVENTATIVE MEASURES

If this is the first time management has sought to deal with this health and safety problem then it will be necessary to devise a strategy with medium and long-term objectives. As a guide it is worth remembering that employers are required under the Health and Safety at Work Act 1974 to provide certain things for their employees. This can provide a framework for devising preventative measures. Employers are required by the Act to provide:

- safe systems of work (working practices);
- safe and healthy workplaces;
- safe and healthy working environments; and
- information, instruction and training.

SAFE SYSTEMS OF WORK

Working practices

In the health care sector the relevant questions about working practices could be:

1. Why is any job done in a particular way?
   (a) Is it because it has always been done that way?
   (b) Has the working method just developed over time or has experience shown that it is the only way to do the job well?
   (c) When decisions are made about working methods is any consideration given to the risk of violence?
   (d) Are staff and trade union representatives consulted?
2. Do certain jobs have to be done by one person working in isolation with the client? Could the job not be done just as well or even more effectively by two people working together at all times?
3. When team discussions take place about the needs of the client is any consideration given at this stage to the health and safety of the staff involved? Do patient care plans not only take account of the care needs of the patient but include an assessment of the likelihood of an aggressive response towards the member of staff?
4. When decisions about the withdrawal of services are made is the risk of resulting violence considered? In long-stay hospitals if the occupational therapy service is cut will this result in a reduction of activities available to clients and the possible increase in boredom and negative reactions?
5. Are clients given information about procedures and timing so that they are less likely to blame the staff for something they do not like or that they find unsatisfactory?
6. Do decisions about staffing levels, staffing rotas and the length of time individuals are exposed to the public take into account the risk of violence?

Decisions about the need for a certain approach such as doubling-up of staff should be made because of the nature of the case and not left to individuals to decide that they need help. Considerations of the risks to staff should be part of the overall management of a client's case.

If the risk cannot be removed then the worker should be removed from the risk or at least his/her exposure to the risk should be reduced. This is accepted as a proper way to deal with other known health and safety problems so why not with the risk of violence from the public in the health care sector?

Staffing levels and hours of work

The HSAC guidance produced for the health services suggests that the following points about staff levels should be considered:

- unpredictable and unremitting work loads lead to fatigue and a diminished ability both to identify early and to subsequently cope with potentially violent situations;
- there should be sufficient flexibility in the provision of staff to adjust levels to meet actual needs;
- there should be adequate cover for nights, weekends and change-over periods between shifts;
- individuals should not be left isolated for long periods nor should junior or inexperienced staff have to cope alone, especially in situations where there is a recognized potential for violence or where patients may take advantage; and
- where there is a well-established risk there should be an agreed number of appropriately qualified staff on duty at any one time.

SAFE WORKPLACES

Some of the questions to ask about the workplace to identify any changes that are necessary could be:

1. The workplace of health care staff will include areas set aside for the public to wait.
   (a) Can these be changed in any way to reduce tension levels ... lighting, decoration, number of seats available, the arrangement of seating, access to refreshments, telephones, etc?
   (b) Can arrangements be made to provide play areas for children?
   (c) Do waiting areas need to be large or would it be helpful to keep people in more human-sized spaces?
2. Could the system for seeing people be changed so that at no time in the day do people feel they are part of a large crowd waiting for very different or scarce services? For example, a GP practice could have a large waiting area with four consulting rooms with surgeries all held at the same time, or it could provide small waiting areas near each consulting room and stagger the times of each surgery

so that the member of the public does not see more than a handful of people or feel part of a crowd.

3. Do interviewing rooms offer the staff a means of easy retreat as well as offering privacy to the client?
4. Are any offices situated away from the mainstream of the activity of the unit, leaving staff to work alone but still accessible to a member of the public?
5. How easy is it for members of the public to wander about the workplace unnoticed and unchecked?
6. Do the public need access to the whole workplace at any time of the day or night?
7. Are any premises more isolated at particular times of the day and night?
8. Are areas between buildings and car parks well-lit at night? Are all lights including those within buildings regularly maintained?
9. Have members of staff been provided with an alarm switch on their desks or in their rooms to enable them to summon help?
    (a) Are these alarms efficiently maintained?
    (b) Has a procedure been established to ensure that help is always forthcoming?

Help may be the arrival of more staff in the area or the involvement of a trained team who can lead a very distressed and angry person to a quiet room where the problem can be dealt with without putting staff at risk or causing more violence among those in the area. If alarms have been fitted is it clearly understood by all staff that they are encouraged to use the alarms when they feel unsure or uncomfortable and that this will not be taken as a sign of weakness?

Staff working in the community and in clients' homes face particular risks that will require a different response from management. Again the risk assessment should highlight any specific measures that need to be taken. On home visits the following questions may be relevant:

• Is there a policy on home visits?
• Is there a need to reassess this, especially with regard to those visits made late at night in isolated areas?
• Which home visits are essential for the care of the client and which could just as well be replaced with visits by the client to the unit?
• What arrangements are made to manage home visits?

The DHSS committee included the following useful checklists on home visits in its report. The first is a home-visit checklist for managers:

1. Are your staff who visit:
    (a) Fully trained in strategies for the prevention of violence?
    (b) Briefed about the area where they work?

(c) Aware of attitudes, traits or mannerisms that can annoy clients, etc.?

(d) Given all available information about the client from all relevant agencies?

2. Have they:
   (a) Understood the importance of previewing cases?
   (b) Left an itinerary?
   (c) Made plans to keep in contact with colleagues?
   (d) The means to contact you – even when the switchboard may not be in use?
   (e) Your home telephone number (and you theirs)?
   (f) A sound grasp of your organization's preventive strategy?
   (g) Authority to arrange an accompanied visit, security escort or use of taxis?

3. Do they:
   (a) Carry forms for reporting incidents?
   (b) Appreciate the need for this procedure?
   (c) Use them?
   (d) Know your attitude to premature termination of interviews?
   (e) Know how to control and defuse potentially violent situations?
   (f) Appreciate their responsibilities for their own safety?
   (g) Understand the provisions for their support by your organization?

The second is a home-visiting checklist for staff who make home visits:

1. Have you:
   (a) Had all the relevant training about violence to staff?
   (b) A sound grasp of **your** unit's safety policy for visitors?
   (c) A clear idea about the area into which **you** are going?
   (d) Carefully previewed today's cases for potential for violence?
   (e) Asked to 'double up', take an escort or use a taxi if unsure?
   (f) Made appointment(s)?
   (g) Left **your** itinerary and expected departure/arrival times?
   (h) Told colleagues, manager, etc. about possible changes of plan?
   (i) Arranged for contact if **your** return is overdue?

2. Do you carry:
   (a) Forms to record and report 'incidents'?
   (b) A personal alarm or radio? Does it work? Is it handy?
   (c) A bag/briefcase, wear an outer uniform or car stickers that suggest **you** have money or drugs with you? Is this wise where **you** are going today/tonight?
   (d) Out-of-hours telephone numbers, etc. to summon help?

3. Can you:
   (a) Be certain **your** attitudes, body language, etc. will not cause trouble?
   (b) Defuse potential problems and manage aggression?

The three 'Vs' of visiting are 'Vet, Verify and Vigilance'.

A SAFE AND HEALTHY WORKING ENVIRONMENT

The work environment includes not only the physical workplace but all aspects of the organization involving relationships between staff; the design of jobs and the management style. Specific questions about the working environment could be:

- Has management made clear by its actions that it takes its responsibilities for the health and safety of employees seriously?
- Does the management style encourage staff to believe that their needs have been taken into account as well as those of the clients?
- Do they know what to do if they are involved in a violent incident?
- Has counselling and support been arranged for those involved in a violent incident and for their colleagues?
- Do they have the confidence that if they call for help it will be provided?
- Can they work easily knowing that they are unlikely to be confronted unexpectedly by an unknown angry member of the public?

INFORMATION, INSTRUCTION AND TRAINING

Under the Management of Health and Safety at Work Regulations employers have a responsibility to provide employees with the information they may need to ensure that they will be able to work without a threat to their health and safety. Training is a support to a preventative policy. It is part of the strategy but can only make a contribution once the risk assessment has been made and preventative measures planned. It is not a substitute for safe systems of work and safe workplaces.

The HSAC guidance (1987) recommended that for all staff working in the area where the risk of violence has been established there should be a short course providing discussion of:

- causes of violence;
- recognition of warning signs;
- relevant interpersonal skills; and
- details of arrangements devised by management.

Although training is not a substitute for other forms of risk assessment it has been shown to decrease the levels of violence. For example, Whittington and Wykes (1993) trained hospital nurses and found that when enough staff on a particular ward had attended there were reductions in the level of violent incidents. In addition, those who will be given responsibility for handling violent or potentially violent people may need an extra course dealing with methods of diffusing aggression and acceptable methods of restraint.

SIMPLE SINGLE SOLUTIONS

Just as there are no blueprints for dealing with the risk of violence at work there are no easy solutions or short-cuts. However, so often when the risk of violence is raised the discussion quickly turns to personal alarms, panic buttons and self-defence training. All these may be useful but not in isolation. There is a real need to ask a series of simple but critical questions about each of these proposed solutions.

Personal alarms

Regarding personal alarms, the following points may be considered:

- How effective are they at preventing violence?
- Will they be heard by anyone who will know what they are and be willing to offer help?
- Will they give the member of staff a false sense of security and cause them to forget any training they have been given on the warning signs of impending violence?
- Are they likely to cause any violence to escalate?
- Are they a cheap and easy way to deal with a complex problem?
- Do they not pass all the responsibility for dealing with violence to the worker?

Panic buttons

The following should be considered before installing panic buttons:

- What happens when they are pressed – will help arrive quickly?
- Will people be encouraged to use them freely or will they be seen as nuisances or incompetents for doing so?

Self-defence training

If there is a policy to train staff in self-defence the following should be considered:

- When is it acceptable to use violence against a client?
- Who will decide the circumstances when it is permissible?
- Will staff be reassured that as long as they follow the agreed rules they will not be disciplined?
- Will this pass all the responsibility from the employer onto the employee?
- Given one needs practice to be effective, where are staff to get this practice?

These issues have also been discussed in Chapter 10.

MONITORING

Monitoring is an essential part of the management of health and safety. It is a process that provides information essential to the proper management of risk. It allows for a check to be made on the effectiveness of any control measures that have been introduced to prevent risk. It will also help management to meet the requirements in the Management of Health and Safety at Work Regulations, to reassess risk if any circumstances change.

Monitoring will allow a check to be made on how a strategy is being implemented in different parts of the organization. It will ensure not only that effective measures are identified but also those that need to be modified or abandoned. It provides information that can only strengthen the confidence of management, staff and trade union representatives that the arrangements made for health and safety are successful.

CONCLUSION

The risk of violence to staff in the health care sector is directly related to the main purpose of the service provided for and on behalf of the community. This determines the jobs that are created and the circumstances in which they have to be performed. There are no obvious easy solutions to preventing and managing the risk but the complexity is no reason for delay or inaction by employers. Many other health and safety problems more easily acknowledged by employers are equally complex.

The management of this health and safety problem requires a multidisciplinary approach involving line management, staff, unions, health and safety specialists, fire and security officers. It is not sufficient to pass this issue on to the security department as if the violence to staff in the health care sector is the same as theft or vandalism of property.

Employees have a right to be healthy and safe at work including being safe from foreseeable incidents of violence. Trade unions have been arguing at least since the early 1980s that violence at work is a legitimate and serious work-related risk for many workers and that employers have legal duties to identify and prevent that risk. The welcome initiatives of the Health and Safety Commission, the HSE and the DHSS Committee have confirmed this. However, unless there is positive action in the workplace, their initiatives will be wasted and there will be more deaths, more injuries and a greater loss of experience, skill and commitment to an essential human service.

The law requires that the risks to the health and safety of employees must be assessed and preventative measures introduced when it is not possible to eliminate the risk. The authoritative advice has been published and, in April 1995, it is likely that acts of physical violence will have to be reported under the proposed Reporting of Injuries Regulations. The experience and empirical data described in this book should be used to create changes that will make for a safer and healthier working life. The need for a commitment and a systematic approach to a serious health and safety problem could not be clearer.

BIBLIOGRAPHY

HSE (1988) *Preventing Violence to Staff*, HSE, London.
HSE (1989) *Violence to Staff*, (free booklet), HSE, London.
HSAC (1987) *Violence to Staff in the Health Service*, London.
DHSS (1988) *Report of the DHSS Advisory Committee on Violence to Staff*, DHSS, London.
Association of Directors of Social Services (1987) *Guidelines and Recommendations to Employers on Violence Against Employees*, ADSS, London.
COHSE (1988) Violence Factsheet, COHSE, London.
COHSE (1989) Model Policy – Following Skelmersdale, COHSE, London.
NALGO (1988) *Violence at Work – Report of the DHSS Advisory Committee on Violence to Staff*, NALGO, London.
NALGO (1992) *Violence at Work – A Preventative Strategy*, NALGO, London.
NUPE (1990) *Survey on Violence to Health Care Staff*, NUPE, London.
NUPE (1991) *Guidelines on Violence in the NHS*, NUPE, London.

NUPE (1993) *Survey on Violence to Health Care Staff*, NUPE, London.
TUC (1988) *Hazards at Work* (Ch. 25), TUC, London, pp. 170–74.
Whittington, R. and Wykes, T. (1993) Violence in psychiatric hospitals: Are certain staff prone to be assaulted? *Journal of Advanced Nursing*, (in press).

Information on professional, trade union and voluntary groups who offer assistance to victims

Trade Union and Professional Organizations: Advice and information for their members

Organization	Address	Telephone No.	Advice and/or assistance provided
COHSE[a]	Glen House, High Street, Banstead, Surrey, SM7 2LH	0737 353322	Information and guidance for branches on preventative strategies; provision of legal advice and support for members involved in violent incidents at work
NALGO[a]	1 Mabledon Place London, WC1H 9AJ	071 388 2366	Information and guidance for branches on preventative strategies; provision of legal advice and support for members involved in violent incidents at work
NUPE[a]	Civic House 20 Grand Depot Road, London, SE18 6SF	081 854 2244	Information and guidance for branches on preventative strategies; provision of legal advice and support for members involved in violent incidents at work; new document on managing violence in the workplace (see Appendix B)

Organization	Address	Telephone No.	Advice and/or assistance provided
Medical Practitioners Union	50 Southwark Street London, SE1 1UN	071 378 2100	Access to legal advice; local support, advice and representation through MSF (the parent organization) and its regional officers
MSF	Park House, 64–66 Wandsworth Common Northside, London, SW18 2SH	081 871 2100 Health and Safety Office: 0279 65811	Produced guidelines on violence at work including model agreements for prevention, staff support etc. in 'Prevention of Violence at Work' 1993 (see Appendix B); local support from branch officials and regional officers including access to legal advice, help with compensation and representation
BMA	BMA House Tavistock Square, London, WC1H 9JP	071 387 4499	Recent document 'Violence at Work', September 1993. Advice on effects and policy
Medical Defence Union	3 Devonshire Place London, W1M 9AE	071 486 6181	Provide advice and informal support following threats, harassment and violence, produced booklets on 'Talking to Patients' and 'Coping with Complaints in General Practice as part of their advice to reduce levels of violence
Royal College of Nursing	20 Cavendish Square, London, W1M 0AB	071 409 3333	Some guidelines for aggression in accident and emergency departments; access to CHAT, supportive helpline for staff; some legal advice available
Royal College of Psychiatrists	17 Belgrave Square, London, SW1X 8PG	071 235 2351	

Organization	Address	Telephone No.	Advice and/or assistance provided
Royal College of Midwives	15 Mansfield Street, London, W1M 0BE	071 580 6523	General guidelines on health and safety; will ensure that employer has done everything to reduce the risks in the environment; will help victims apply for compensation
British Association of Social Workers	16 Kent Street, Birmingham, B5 6RD	021 622 3911	Advice, support and representation (e.g. to tribunals or employers); also access to legal advice
British Psychological Society	48 Princess Road East, Leicester, LE1 7DR	0533 549568	Division of Clinical Psychology has produced a guidance document called 'Prevention and Management of Violence at Work' (BPS, 1992)
General Medical Council	44 Hallam Street, London, W1N 6AE	071 580 7642	General advice contained in 'Professional Conduct and Discipline: Fitness to Practice'
Health Visitors Association	50 Southwark Street, London, SE1 1UN	071 378 7255	New guidelines on procedures for violence at work for health authorities and trusts; has information on how to diffuse situation; suggests on-site support for staff provided by employer

[a] All three unions have now amalgamated and are called UNISON.

Voluntary Organizations

Organization	Address	Telephone No.	Advice provided
National Association of Victim Support Schemes	Cranmer House, 39 Brixton Road, London, SW9 6DZ	071 735 9166	The heaquarters of a national network of volunteer counsellors organized in local areas; ring for your nearest branch; counsellors will provide emotional and practical support
Rape Crisis	PO Box 69, London, WC1X 9NJ	Counselling no.: 071 837 1600 Office no: 071 916 5466	Will provide immediate advice following rape or sexual assault
WASH (Women Against Sexual Harassment)	312 The Chandlery, 50 Westminster Bridge Road, London, SE1 7QY	071 721 7592 Information: 061 833 9244	Provide legal advice, general advice, on coping strategies and counselling on sexual harassment
City Centre	32–35 Featherstone Street, London, EC1Y 8QX	071 608 1338	Informal advice, support and counselling about sexual harassment

Compensation and Legal Advice

Organization	Address	Telephone No.	What do they provide?
Criminal Injuries Compensation Board	Blythswood House, 200 West Regent Street, Glasgow, G2 4SW	041 221 0945	Advice on making applications for compensation for physical and psychological injury; claims have to be over £1000 (see Chapter 8 for details)
Central Office of the Industrial Tribunals (for England and Wales)	100 Southgate Street, Bury St Edmunds, Suffolk, IP33 2AQ	0284 762300	Advice on compensation and tribunals that can assess whether, for instance, sexual harassment has occurred; ask for form IT1
Central Office of the Industrial Tribunals (for Scotland)	St Andrew House, 141 West Nile Street, Glasgow, G1 2RU	041 331 1601	Advice on compensation and tribunals that can assess whether, for instance, sexual harassment has occurred; ask for form IT1
Office of the Industrial Tribunals and the Fair Employment Tribunal (for Northern Ireland)	Long Bridge House, 20–25 Waring Street, Belfast, BT1 2EB	0232 327666	Advice on compensation and tribunals that can assess whether, for instance, sexual harassment has occurred; ask for form IT1
National Association of Citizens Advice Bureaux	115 Pentonville Road, London N1 9LZ (or look in the phone book for your local office)	071 833 2181	General advice on who you should contact and how to do it
Law Centres Federation	Duchess House, Warren Street, London W1P 5DA (or look up your local office in the phone book)	071 387 8570	The federation itself cannot give advice but can put you in touch with your local office who will be able to help

Other help for the victims of violence

Organization	Address	Telephone no.	What do they provide?
Psychologists	Either in your local general practice or in your local hospital		Contact through your general practitioner who will refer you on to the appropriate source; provide treatment of victims' psychological problems
Occupational Health	In your employer's list of services		Contact directly; usually offer crisis support but will refer on to other sources if necessary
Service for Sick Doctors		071 935 5982	Will put doctors, their colleagues and spouses in touch with local advisors who will provide support and advice following an incident at work
CHAT	At the RCN (see page 248)	071 409 3333	Telephone advice on psychological and other problems

Bibliography

BASIC GUIDES ON VIOLENCE AT WORK

Breakwell, G. (1989) *Facing Physical Violence*, British Psychological Association, London.

British Association of Social Workers (1988) *Violence to Social Workers*, BASW, Birmingham.

Brown, R., Bute, S. and Ford, P. (1986) *Social Workers at Risk. The Prevention and Management of Violence*, BASW, London.

Curtis, L. (1993) *Making Advances: What You Can Do About Sexual Harrassment At Work*, BBC Books, London.

Department of Employment (1992) *Sexual Harassment in the Workplace: A Guide for Employers*, Department of Employment, London.

Department of Employment (1993) *Sexual Harassment in the Workplace: Facts Employees Should Know.* Department of Employment, London.

Department of Health (1988) *Violence to Staff: Report of the DHSS Advisory Committee on Violence to Staff*, HMSO, London.

HSAC (1987) *Violence to Staff in the Health Services*, HMSO, London.

Institute of Personnel Management (1992) *Statement on Harassment at Work*, IPM, London.

Lamplugh, D. (1988) *Beating Aggression. A Practical Guide for the Working Woman*, Weidenfeld and Nicolson, London.

Lion, J.R. and Reid, W.H. (1983) *Assaults in Psychiatric Facilities.* Grune and Stratton, London.

Poyner, B. and Warne, C. (1986) *Violence to Staff: A Basis for Assessment and Prevention.* HSE, London.

Poyner, B. and Warne, C. (1988) *Preventing Violence to Staff.* HSE/Tavistock Institute for Human Relations, London.

Rubenstein, M. (1992) *Preventing and Remedying Sexual Harassment at Work*, Industrial Relations Services, London.

Wilson, J. and Raphael, B. (1993) *International Handbook of Traumatic Stress Syndromes*. Plenum, London.

THE UNDERLYING CAUSES OF VIOLENCE

Felson, R. and Tedeschi, J. (eds) (1993) *Aggression and Violence*, American Psychological Association, Washington.
Howells, K. and Hollin, C. (eds) (1989) *Clinical Approaches to Violence*, John Wiley, Chichester.
Toch, H. (1992) *Violent Men*, American Psychological Association, Washington.

TRAINING INFORMATION

Harris, A., Wykes, T., Brisby, T. *et al.* (1993) *Prevention and Management of Violence in General Practice*. Lambeth, Southwark and Lewisham FHSA, London.
Surrey County Council (1991) *Safe and Secure*, (training manual). Surrey County Council, Guildford.

TREATMENT OF PERPETRATORS

Roth, L. (1987) *Clinical Treatment of the Violent Person*, Guilford Press, New York.

TREATMENT OF VICTIMS

Bard, M. and Sangrey, D. (eds) (1986) *The Crime Victim's Handbook*, 2nd edn, Brunner/Mazel, New York.
Figley, C. (ed) (1985) *Trauma and its Wake: The Study and Treatment of Post-Traumatic Stress Disorder*, Brunner/Mazel, New York.
Miers, D. (1990) *Compensation for Criminal Injuries*, Butterworths, London.
Ochberg, F. (ed.) (1987) *Post-Traumatic Therapy and the Victims of Violence*, Brunner/Mazel, New York.
Payne, R. and Firth-Cozens, J. (1987) *Stress in Health Care Professionals*, John Wiley, Chichester.

Index

Page numbers in **bold** type refer to the list of support services and their addresses in Appendix A. n after a page number refers to a footnote.